Dear Julie,

Trust God

and

Buy Broccoli

Written by:

Blissings! Gerri

Gerri Helms

*Our miracles are out there,
if our hearts are open to
receive them!*

Trust God and Buy Broccoli

Published by:
MP Press, A division of
Femme Osage Publishing
1301 Colby Drive
Saint Peters, Missouri, USA 63376
FemmeOsagePublishing.com
Publisher@FemmeOsagePublishing.com

Printed in the United States of America

ISBN: 978-1-934509-05-0

Library of Congress Control Number: 2007931750

First Printing 2007

Author Contact:
Gerri Helms
LifeCoachGerri@aol.com
www.lifecoachgerri.com

What people are saying about

Trust God and Buy Broccoli

"*Trust God and Buy Broccoli* will not disappoint anyone who can relate to the concept of 'food addiction.' Gerri does a great job of conveying, up close and personal, what it's like to struggle with the tyranny of the most common eating disorder of all - food addiction. The reader will not be left only with a story about the problem, but be offered a chance to understand the solution."

Marty Lerner, Ph.D., Executive Director
Milestones Eating Disorders Program
www.milestonesprogram.org

"Gerri writes with honesty and wit, and it's obvious she lives what she writes. This is an excellent addition to the recovery literature for those with binge eating disorder. It contains practical applications of recovery theory to ordinary life situations. It's based soundly in research theory, while being down to earth and pragmatic. A great book for clients struggling with how to begin or continue the drastic change of lifestyle needed to lose and maintain a large amount of weight."

Cindyellen Robinson, LADC, LCMHC
The Adams Center for Mind and Body
www.theadamscenter.com

"This personal confession offers practical advice, particularly to persons with eating disorders. But the book applies to anyone with addictive, compulsive behaviors (all of us!), The reader is invited to notice the feeling driving the unbalanced behavior and to trust God. And Gerri's life encourages us - *freedom from* enslavement does bring *freedom for* relationship with self, others and God."

Fr. Bill Creed, SJ
Chicago IL
www.ignatianspiritualityproject.org

"Reading this book, I was astounded that someone knew the depths of my despair. I found it to be written with brutal honesty, hilarious wit, and best of all, clear direction. I felt I finally had an ally, that maybe I could overcome compulsive overeating by taking the steps outlined between the covers. I will buy this book for everyone I know that is suffering from compulsive overeating. I ate this book up!"

Jennifer J. Sampson
West Palm Beach, FL

"Hope ... That is what I get with each page of this book. How can I express my gratitude for a book that could easily be entitled, *Dear Mary*? I thank you for the bottom of my heart for giving me hope to fight yet another day through my own struggle with this deadly disease. This book is truly inspired by God through author Gerri Helms."
Mary Dominguez
Clermont, FL

"It is obvious that this author knows what she is talking about. I believe this wonderful book will help many who struggle with an eating disorder."
Rene Poe, LCDC
Granbury, Texas

"Gerri has summarized in this magnificent book, years of success, many miles and milestones of any diet survivor's journey. As an emotional eating survivor, I am confident this book will help many of us who are still on the healing path. Thank you for this great work, Coach Gerri."
Mazen S. Alzogbi
Life Coach
Saudi Arabia

What people are saying about

Life Coach Gerri Helms

"We are delighted to have Life Coach Gerri Helms as an ACORN associate. She shares her proven experience on how to functionally deal with eating while socializing, in restaurants, at work, and in other challenging situations for newly recovered individuals. Many of our clients have benefited from working with Gerri."

Phil Werdell, M.A.
Acorn Food Dependency Recovery Svcs
www.foodaddiction.com

"Gerri Helms is one of those rare people who 'walks the talk.' When I called Gerri I was 100 pounds overweight, in complete despair of ever losing even an ounce, and believing I was a hopeless failure in all areas of my life. In the six short months I have been working with her, I have lost 31 pounds, still losing, and confident I will succeed. However, more importantly, Gerri helps me dig through and sort out the hopes and dreams I have put on hold or given up on throughout my life, and even more amazing, dream new ones! Gerri encourages me, helps me celebrate ALL accomplishments, and holds me accountable. She has the wonderful ability to cut through much of my unnecessary chatter, read in between the lines, and focus on what I should really be working on. Gerri is a wonderful life coach, and I know she will soar to the heights of her profession. I'm thrilled to be on the journey with her."

Elizabeth R
Middle School English Teacher
California

"Gerri Helms, Life Coach is an incredible woman. Since I have known her both professionally and personally I have seen her commitment to grow, learn, build a successful coaching practice, send out daily musings and fulfill her dream...write a book. Gerri is talented, creative and a down to earth woman who you can trust to be there when the going get rough. I am thrill and so excited for you, Ger...the best is yet to come. "

Lorraine Edey, LCSW, PhD
Life/Relationship Coach
www.coachinginspirations.com

"I never knew before I met Gerri that God could speak to me through those little green florets called broccoli! There is no place, whether in a store, or my own home, that when I see broccoli I don't think of the wonderful influence Gerri Helms has had

on my life! She is my coach and mentor! Her book is bound to be a best seller."
    Linda R
    Cambridge City
    Indiana

"Through humor, personal experience and generosity, Gerri has inspired and educated our employees. She is always willing to offer assistance."
    Kim Brooks
    Human Resource Manager
    DiPasqua, Enterprises
    Orlando, FL.
    subwaydipasqua.com

"Gerri is a strong, enthusiastic personality without being just a "cheerleader". She has walked through some very deep valleys of her own and has emerged into a great life. As my life coach, she has held my hand while I guided myself through uncharted territories and gave me the confidence in myself that I really needed at that time. I will always feel that I could not have come through some of these times as successfully without her support."
    Rudine B
    Titusville, FL

"Starting a new venture is always like jumping into the unknown. That's what it felt like when I finally agreed to "work with a coach." Gerri has been awesome. She listens, she prods, she suggests and she guides. Gerri is all about tackling the well-being of the whole person. Setting goals is never easy and certainly trying to arrive at the goals can sometimes be more than difficult. This coaching experience has taught me to set reasonable goals and to be mindful about what I do and say. I can honestly say that after a few months of coaching, Gerri has helped me name the goals that I would like for myself and has shown me that they are obtainable."

Dorie
Orlando, FL

Dedication

To my friends around the world, who have sent me broccoli jokes and stories. The support of people who understand food addiction helped me to trust God first. *Trust God and Buy Broccoli* is dedicated to you

To David, my supportive and loving husband, thank you and I love you.

I am grateful beyond words that this whole adventure called my life is no longer about being face first in a pizza.

If you have tried dieting and lost weight, but can't maintain the loss, this book is for you. I am one of you. The last time my weight exceeded two hundred pounds, I was desperate for something, anything, to work.

Looking back, perhaps any weight loss plan would have worked, except there were thing about myself that I didn't know. Now I understand that I am addicted to certain foods, and much like a cocaine addict, when these foods are ingested, I cannot stop eating.

Originally, this was a cookbook, but it evolved into sharing my lifestyle changes for people who may also have trouble keeping off excess pounds. I am not a nutritionist or a doctor. My area of expertise comes from years of battling morbid obesity and failed diets. I could never hit goal weight, a healthy, normal weight, in any program I tried. When I got close, one celebration with food would bring back the bingeing.

Since 1993, I have maintained a weight loss of over one hundred pounds. Perhaps the techniques and lifestyle changes that work for me will work for you too.

Acknowledgements

Editor – Pam Strickland

Pam Strickland is a widely published essayist and journalist for both regional and national publications writing on politics, social justice, religion, health and family. Currently adjunct teaching at her undergraduate alma mater, the University of Tennessee, Strickland is co- author of the upper elementary fiction book, Under One Flag: A Year at Rohwer by August House Publishing, which is a 2006 Historic Preservation Book Prize nominee. She has also done editing for August House and others.

Cover Design - 'Cyanotype Book Architects' http://www.cyanotype.ca/

Table of Contents

Chapter One
Once Upon a Time

It was just another ordinary night in the spring of 1993. I was driving home from my job as a corporate sales manager at a nice hotel, just off International Drive in Orlando. I stopped at the 7-Eleven near Wet and Wild, and bought two Dove ice cream bars and inhaled them before I reached the McDonald's on Kirkman Road. Next was a large milkshake, a quarter-pound burger, and a large order of French fries. I had to really shove those down because there was only a few miles between there and home.

The wrappers and bags joined my many other binge containers under the front seat of my car. The evidence was hidden as I approached the top of our street, and my nightly fantasy began again.

I pictured my handsome husband waiting for me at the door, our two-point-five children nestled in bed while the *Theme From Love* Story played in my head. We'd have cocktails and a gourmet dinner and make mad, passionate love all evening.

Reality? There were no children. That handsome husband was sprawled on the couch watching *Star Trek*, nursing his hangover from the night before and couldn't have cared less that I was home. Trying to make the fantasy real, I went to hug him, but he held my wrists, preventing me from getting my arms around him. Disgust and contempt were reflected on his face. All that food from the trip home did not take away the pain. My heart ached as I walked to the bedroom to change.

The wardrobe selection had dwindled down to one super sized, threadbare housecoat. As I disrobed, I looked in the mirror and saw that I had chocolate on my face from the ice cream. Ketchup had dripped on my business suit lapel; I was a mess. My teeth were not clean, for I only brushed them occasionally. I had body odor -- couldn't reach all the parts when I did bathe, which also wasn't daily. Too much trouble. I was so depressed that everything but eating was too much trouble.

Meanwhile, my husband had gone to bed to sleep off his hangover for a return to work that evening. Did I mention that he was a bartender in a nude bar? Well, he was. As he slept, I cooked and ate a whole chicken and a box of pasta loaded with butter, sat down on the couch and thought my stomach would burst wide open. It hurt so bad. I comforted myself with pretzels. I was at my lowest.

Sometime in there my husband left for work. The drapes were drawn, the house dark. I couldn't think of a single person to call. There was only me and my best friend, food, who had also turned on me. I thought of ways to kill myself.

Maybe I could find all the pills we had in the house: aspirin, diet pills, sleeping pills, cold tablets. I could take them all, wash them down with scotch whiskey and that would do it. Or would it? No, wait, could I slit my wrists? No, that would hurt too much. My husband had a gun. Oh. no, that would be too terrible for my family.

In quiet desperation, I cried out to a God that I didn't believe in and asked Him to help me. He did – I passed out.

How had it come to this? How did life get this bad?

I wasn't fat as a kid. Second in a family of six, sandwiched in between two brothers, I was an active tomboy who played hard. I swam competitively, was a flag twirler in my high school band, and rode my bike everywhere.

However, at four years old, I was already stealing candy, and whenever I could get away with it, ate more than my share. Probably all the activity kept me from being overweight.

My senior year in high school, I had surgery for a knee injury, and the evidence of my overeating surfaced for the first time. I was seventeen and gaining weight rapidly.

That summer, as the weight went up, my self-esteem went down. Dates were few and far between. If a fellow asked, I accepted and overeating was temporarily replaced with alcohol. Now, along with being fat, I was drinking too much too. How would

I ever meet a nice guy? I just had to lose weight.

So my dieting career began with Aydes candies. Remember them? Take one or two with a cup of hot tea. I always ate more than two, but lost weight anyway.

Thus began a thirty-year stint of yo-yo dieting. At age eighteen, when my first husband proposed to me I was a size sixteen. By April of the following year, I fit into a size ten wedding gown.

I have gone over two hundred pounds three times in my twenty-five year eating career. The last time, when I hit two hundred forty eight, I just quit weighing myself and went uptwo more dress sizes to a plus size twenty-four, so I don't really know my exact top weight.

In January of 1993, I had begun to experience heart palpitations. Both my mother and oldest brother have diabetes, and I feared that would be next. My doctor said I was borderline. At forty-three years old, my joints hurt and my feet stung when they hit the floor in the morning. The cardiologist told me if I didn't do something about my weight, I probably would not see my fiftieth birthday.

So I went back to one of the popular diet clubs. I thought, "This time, I'll prepay for a whole year. Yeah, that will do it." When I left, I went straight to the closest frozen yogurt shop and binged. Again. I thought, "Hell, if I'm gonna die at fifty, I may as well enjoy myself." Food, food, food. That's what my life had narrowed down to. Just me and food.

Shortly after my brush with suicide, a friend from work who recognized my depression gave me a book to read about food addiction. For the first time in my life, it seemed like somebody understood what was going on with me. That book really changed how I thought about food.

I grabbed onto the principles in that book and I've never looked back. I wrote down what happened that horrible night when I nearly killed myself and carried that piece of paper in my pocket for nearly a year, until it finally went through the washing machine. Whenever a pizza seemed like a good idea, I'd take that paper out and read it. Today it is deeply ingrained in my brain.

That is my reality of returning to exc
food. I'll probably kill myself.

While that book really launched a who
new way of eating for me, as time went on
I discovered more about myself and why I
ate the way I did. As my weight went down,
my self-esteem went up. My husband and
I divorced. I moved out on my own for the
first time in my life and didn't overeat to
deal with all the new experiences. I learned
how to deal with life without having to resort to excess food.

Perhaps you could say I have twenty-five
years of unsuccessful dieting to my credit.
Prior to this success with weight loss, I had
tried so many diets. Atkins, Stillman, and
The Dolly Parton Diet. The T-Factor, high
protein, low fat, low protein, high fat. I used
diet pills, protein shakes, peed on a stick
that was supposed to turn purple for ke-
tosis or some nonsense like that. Life was
either dieting or bingeing. No normal eating
for over twenty-five years.

I am so grateful today for this sane life I
live. Some people who eat like me possibly
have chemical imbalances and may even
need medication to reverse it. I was lucky,

, how I ate really had a huge
y cravings. I rarely experience
y more. The compulsion to over
etty much been lifted. Best of all,
the excess weight and have kept it
ever was able to do that in the past.
says something about the changes I
e made.

Oh, I have my days when I'd like to really rip into food, but they are few and far between. When the compulsion hits, I no longer need to act on it. Period.

Chapter Two
Are You Really Ready?

There are many ways to lose weight, but if you aren't ready, you aren't ready. Unless you are really ready to make changes in your life and thinking, your chances for success are not likely. Honestly, many people want to lose weight, but don't want to do the work to make it happen. I know, I was once there.

I did not get to two hundred forty eight overnight. It took a massive amount of work. It takes a massive amount of work to become morbidly obese. It takes a massive amount of work to stay morbidly obese. In order to lose weight, I had to put as much, if not more energy into weight loss as I did into the weight gain. There just aren't any easy formulas or shortcuts.

Starving won't do it either. I tried that. For me it actually had an opposite effect from what I wanted to accomplish. My body must have some sort of self preservation mode to protect itself from me. After a few days of fasting, the weight loss would totally stall and I'd return to overeating.

Toward the end of my eating career, I'd try to go on a very strict plan of five hundred calories and five grams of fat a day. Looking back, I can see how crazy that is, but I really, really wanted it to work. I wanted to starve for a few days and go down three or four dress sizes. Lose fifty pounds. Overnight.

It doesn't work that way. Sure, the first day or two, there'd be a significant downward slide on the scale. That would give me the incentive to do another day. After a few days, the scale would stop going down. I'd get discouraged and binge. Then the scale would start going up again. In fact, all the diets I went on had a similar pattern -- quick drop in weight followed by a stall period and then return to overeating.

The scale became the god of my understanding. It did. It ruled my life. If the numbers went down, I'd be thrilled. That would set the tone for the day. It didn't necessarily make sense.

Sometimes the downward slide gave me incentive to diet another day. More often, it gave me permission for a little treat. That treat inevitably lead to a second treat. Within days, the scale would show an upward trend, and I'd get discouraged. My thoughts, "This diet isn't working." So, out the window it went.

I could completely negate a treat's caloric impact if it were fat-free. There was a period where I went to the gym nearly every day on an empty stomach, rode a stationary bike at a level six for over an hour. My legs were so weak, I could barely walk to the locker room. On the way to work, I'd stop to pick up a dozen fat-free muffins.

One muffin would lead to another, and then another. I'd arrive at work with half a dozen muffins. Strangely enough, those five or six I ate on the way to the office didn't count. The fat-free negated the caloric content. Right? Doesn't it? Butter on a fat-free muffin didn't count either. Total denial: Don't Even Notice I Am Lying.

11

So, of course, the exercise did not result in weight loss. I had a trainer at the time who couldn't understand why I was gaining. He suggested a low-fat diet. I probably didn't even look at the diet. I just looked for fat-free foods and over ate those.

That thinking had to change if I wanted permanent weight loss. I also had to let go of daily scale hopping. That was really hard. How could I measure the success of my newest diet without my old buddy, Mr. Scale?

With my food plan geared to weight loss, I weighed myself once a month. Wow, was that a radical concept for me. Initially, I had my then-husband hide the scale. It was too hard to go in the bathroom, look at it every day and not hop on.

The second thing I did was to find a reasonable plan of eating that encompassed a balanced amount of carbohydrates proteins, fats, vegetables. More importantly, it eliminated foods that triggered binges. They don't call 'em trigger foods for nothing – for me eating one is like putting a gun to my head.

My list of trigger foods has changed over time. It will probably change again as my circumstances change. One thing that will not change, however, is that I cannot add the foods back that trigger bingeing. The list is sacred to me. I am open to adding food to it, if it becomes a problem, but once it's on, it's on.

There are no quick fixes either. I've seen many people have the surgical cure, and after great weight loss return to morbid obesity. They forgot to change the way they think, so it was inevitable they found their way back to old eating patterns. My personal opinion on gastic bypass surgery is neutral. Some may need it for health reasons. But unless that person changes how they think, the surgery may not have a lasting effect.

How could I go through life, denying myself those wonderful treats, some ask? That thinking had to change. Treats are tricks. They trick me into believing that one bite won't hurt. It does. It does. It does. Period.

I also had to re-think my relationship to food in general. It is not a solution to my problems, not ever. If the house is on fire, a dozen cream-filled donuts will not put out a fire. I need to call 9-1-1 like everybody else. Food will not make my husband come home on time, or take away pre-nuptial anxiety. How did other people deal with life without a pizza? Or two? Or three? That's what I had to learn.

Another important concept for me is that my results are better if I use the team method. I must align myself with others who want a healthy, normal-sized body and clear mind. That meant taking a vacation from binge buddies. I lost contact with some friends from the past. Our common interest was bingeing, and I wasn't doing that any more. One friend in particular got very angry with me when I changed my lifestyle.

We had been Friday night binge buddies for years, starting out at happy hour eating all the free food and washing it down with two-for-one drinks. Then it was off to dinner, usually high-carb, high-fat fare. And, of course, polish that off with a huge dessert.

She was not ready to make a lifestyle change and so we went our separate ways. That was hard. I really missed her; I still do.

I truly got ready for change when the pain of overeating was worse than the idea of going without. I was so sick of not being able to do things. I hated to shop for clothes. The selection was not very fashionable in the plus size shops. I didn't feel good -- short of breath all the time, aching joints, and, of course, stomach aches.

I isolated, needing time alone to eat in peace. I was often embarrassed by crude remarks from people. Once in the grocery store, a little kid shouted about my very large posterior:

"Mommie, look at that lady's hiney. It's so biiiiiiiiigggggggggg."

I don't know who was more humiliated, me or that poor mommie. I was dying inside, but not knowing how to break out of that crazy cycle of eating. I went home from that grocery trip and binged. Again.

Once I sat on someone's toilet seat and cracked it. I hurt my back at a picnic when the chair I was sitting in collapsed. And then there was the time a stewardess on a plane announced loudly that the lady in row six needed a seat belt extender. Me? A seat belt extender? No. No. No. Not me. I don't need a seat belt extender. That would have meant I was fat. Sure, I had a little problem with food, but, no, I wasn't fat enough for a seat belt extender.

I tugged with all my might and got that unforgiving seatbelt fastened without the extender. Thank God. I would have died from embarrassment. My legs, however, were in terrible pain by the time we landed. I could hardly stand up and didn't think walking off the plane was possible. So, I didn't fly again for many years.

And, I've always had a passion for sports cars. I owned a 1987 Pontiac Fiero, but had to trade it in on a four-door sedan because I couldn't get my large stomach beneath the steering wheel without marking my clothing. That was a very sad day in my life. Excess food was slowly taking away everything I loved.

What made me ready? It was that friend who presented me with the book *Food Addiction, The Body Knows*, by Kay Sheppard that contained concepts I had not ever considered. I am grateful beyond words.

I thought, "Somebody finally understands me, understands how I think, why I do this." It really was the catalyst for changing my life.

So, if you too are really, really ready, hang on to your hat for the ride of your life. A life without excess food. Now don't forget, this isn't a cure-all. It is going to take a lot of work, especially in the beginning. But I promise, it gets easier. And life becomes more fun.

Some of the concepts presented here may seem far fetched, but you know what? They've worked for me. I was really ready, and it worked. I am maintaining this normal body size now for over fourteen years. And you? What have you got to lose? Maybe just a few pounds, or maybe over one hundred pounds. I hope you find an answer in these pages.

Chapter 2

Chapter Three
Diets Don't Work

First off, let me say again that I am not a health care professional. I have no training in medicine or nutrition. My experience comes from nearly thirty years of failed diets. It was only after experiencing, time and time again, what didn't work, that I was able to find something that would work.

It seemed to me that most people who had success with diets also had a book or something; guidelines on how to deal with their life without using food as a crutch. So I tried the books. Every time a new diet book came out, I tried it.

Although initially I was successful at the diet centers and weight loss programs, there'd inevitably come a day when the diet would go out the window. Then I'd be face first in a plate of spaghetti. Ultimately, each diet would result in a weight gain. I would get within a pound or two of hitting goal weight and then fall back into my old eating habits. Why was that?

I'd get close to the goal and celebrate with food. That would be the catalyst that threw me back to the old eating habits, which ultimately lead to morbid obesity. This was a pattern with me. There were at least three or four times that I went to the diet clubs, only to fail again. I felt hopeless in my inability to break that cycle.

At the age of forty-three, more than one hundred pounds over a healthy weight for me, I stopped dieting and changed my life. Not only did I lose that one hundred pounds of excess weight, but also have kept it off ever since. I now am equipped with information about myself that I use as a guideline for living, without excess foods.

Certain foods set up a craving in me and once ingested, it seems I cannot stop eating. I have not eaten foods prepared with flour and sugar since 1993. In my fifth year of this way of eating I discovered that wheat exacerbates a ringing in my ears and purposely haven't eaten wheat since 1998.

Perhaps this is not applicable to you. But something leads you back to eating the way you did prior to the most recent failed diet. What is that for you ? Sugar? Fat? Processed foods? Sweets? Snack foods? Fast foods? Only you can answer this honestly for yourself.

It seems that many of us have trouble with combinations of fat, sugar, and flour. Some high salt foods are difficult for me to control too.

Are you attracted to rattly bags? You know those foods such as chips, pretzels, cookies, and candy bars. Most lack nutritional value and lead to recreational or emotional eating, rather than mindful, healthy eating. They are not conducive to permanent weight loss.

Today I know there is a functional way to stick to a good plan of eating. The diet clubs hand us the diets. The diet books tell us what to eat. But no one really tells us how to live out there in the real world with people who aren't food addicts. Through trial and error on how to maintain my style of eating, I've learned a number of techniques that support a permanent weight loss and being part of society.

The first thing I had to do was change my thinking and priorities, to give up the diet mentality. Today I follow my plan of eating as if my life depends on it. It does. Morbid obesity is a critical disease.

My food plan is my meds. When a doctor prescribes medicine for an illness, I don't take too much or too little, nor do I take any that isn't prescribed for me. This school of thought has proven effective for me.

In addition to my food plan, I abstain from those trigger foods – the ones that when I start eating them, I cannot stop or I find that the next day, I'm craving them. Are there certain foods that cause problems like that for you? Perhaps you'd be better off without them.

You can probably follow any diet if you do not have food addiction problems with certain foods. But if you've reached a critical level like me, it is vital to abstain from any foods that set up a binge. It may take a few days of craving to determine what those foods are for you.

When I watch how my husband David eats, I know that he is not afflicted with food sensitivities like me. Nor does he go bonkers when he eats a little of the foods that I abstain from. I call him a normie. What he can do with food just baffles me. Food does not have the same effect on him as it does on me.

When we first got married in 2001, I wanted to be a good wife, so I started baking for Dave. He'd come home to delicious cakes, pies, and cookies. I didn't eat them, but maybe I was enjoying those sweets vicariously. He gained a few pounds and asked me to stop baking so much. Then he went on one of those low-carb diets for a while, just so his pants would fit comfortably again.

Still wanting to be a good wife, I read up on his diet and prepared the foods he could eat, mostly proteins. One night he stopped eating right in the middle of a steak.

"What's wrong with the steak?"

"Nothing."

"Well, why'd you stop eating it?"

"I'm full."

"But on that diet, it says that you can eat as much as you can."

"No, Honey … it says, 'eat as much as you care to', and that's all I care to eat."

"Oh."

One year, he bought the candy for the trick-or-treaters on Halloween. You know, those little bite-sized Tootsie Rolls? For someone like me, why bother?

After all the kids had come and gone, he took one of those little Tootsie Rolls, about the size of the end of my pinkie, and he bit it in half. Then he wrapped up the other half. That amazed me. I could never eat a bite of a tootsie roll; I'd pretty much need that whole bag.

So, I asked, "What are you doing?" He said he just wanted the taste, so he'd save the other piece for later. Amazing. That whole concept was lost on me. I left that stupid half piece of Tootsie Roll on the counter to see when later actually was. After about a month, I threw it away. He never asked about it.

See, I just don't get that concept, stop when full. Stuffed I know, full is illusive to me. So for the most part, I weigh and measure the majority of my meals. That works for me.

I believe my eyes are broken, and I can't just eyeball stuff. I have no idea what full means. Stuffed, yes, but full, no.

When I eat certain foods, I can't stop thinking about them. Take cookies for instance. Dave can have a package of cookies in the house for weeks. He's thrown them out because they got stale. Well, first I would never have let them get stale. If I did find some stale cookies, it never bothered me if I was in need of a cookie fix. But that's besides the point. I know today that I cannot eat a cookie. If I don't eat a cookie, I can't eat a whole bag. Or two.

Those people who say, "One bite won't hurt." Well, it will hurt me. If I've had one cookie, the darn things start talking to me from the pantry. They'll chat with me until I've eaten the whole bag. If I don't eat the first one, they can sit up there and keep their mouth shut.

When Dave and I got married, we had so much stuff, you know? There was his stuff and my stuff. There was his kid's stuff and then we got our stuff. The kitchen became an obstacle course of stuff.

I went on a quest to rid us of duplicates and simplify the kitchen. Dave likes gadgets, so we also have every modern convenience known to humanity in the kitchen. At least it seems that way.

I found this one weird thing, asked him what it was and he said it was a chip clip. A chip clip? What does one do with a chip clip? I'm trying to picture eating a potato chip with that contraption, when he tells me it is used to keep the bag of chips closed so they stay fresh for the next time. Next time? What next time?

"You mean the bag's not the snack?"

He just looked at me in total amazement. "No Honey, the bag's not the snack."

"Oh."

So this simple concept is that if I don't eat a piece of pizza, I cannot eat a whole pie or two. Oh, my, the times I've had delivery men come to the door with the two pizzas, and I've hollered out, "Hey everybody, the pizzas are here." I was home alone. I could eat two pizzas in an evening, no sweat.

Popcorn's another one. We'd go to the movie and I'd get one of those giant popcorns, the one where you need to take out a second mortgage on your home to buy it. Oh, and money was never an issue when I wanted food.

So I'd get these humongous buckets of popcorn, eat the whole thing, and wish for more. And if you were with me? Don't even think of sticking your hand in my popcorn. I'd have ripped your arm right out at the shoulder. I was self-centered to the max when I was in the midst of a bucket of popcorn. Do you know that I never realized that music plays in the background of most movies until I stopped eating popcorn? Amazing.

My list of problem foods:
- Flour
- Sugar
- Wheat
- Things that come in a bag that rattles (*rattly bag foods*)
- Popcorn
- Sugar-free ice cream or yogurt
- Protein Bars
- Nuts

- Crab salad *(that one is weird. I can eat mayo and I can eat crab but put them together and they rent space in my head) It happens with chicken, shrimp and eggs ... almost any food that is mixed with mayonnaise.*
- Caffeine *(I found that when I have regular coffee, the next day I crave volume)*
- Sugar-free Cool Whip *(I've never had sugar-free Cool Whip but it talks to me in the fridge, so I put it on the list and now it doesn't bother me)*

I'm willing to add foods to this list if they become a problem. As I said earlier, I also don't eat wheat.

I actually got to meet Kay Sheppard, and she challenged me to give up wheat as she considered it an addictive food. I'd been having maybe a bowl of shredded wheat (and I wasn't jonesing for that in-between meals), cream of wheat or Grape Nuts cereal occasionally.

I did not think wheat addiction was a problem, but I agreed I wouldn't eat it for one month. Basically, I thought I'd show Kay Sheppard that it really wasn't addictive for me. Within a few days, there was a marked decrease in the ringing in my ears. Now, if I accidentally get some wheat in a restaurant, I can always tell. My ears ring louder.

In my thinking, there are no cookie-cutter problem foods, although I see many people having trouble with sugar, flour or processed foods like I do. In my estimation, total honesty in this area is critical to permanent weight loss.

I've been on many diets in my bingeing career. I bet you have too, otherwise you'd not be reading this book. Diets all work for a time, but then that fatal day came when I'd reward myself. Next thing you'd know, I'd be trying to get the zipper up on a size sixteen pair of jeans, thinking, "Wait, I'm a size eight." It happens that fast for me. When I was in my late thirties, I once gained nearly a hundred pounds over a summer.

I live a spiritual life now too. When I ask God for help, I get it. Of course, He's not going to the grocery store for me. Or if I wait until I've got an ice cream cone inches from my mouth, odds are fairly good I won't hear Him suggest that it's a bad idea.

It's not really about broccoli, you know. It's about doing the footwork. I believe we all have the answers deep inside of ourselves, and I hope you can reach inside to find what it is for you and achieve permanent weight loss. My plan of eating to lose weight is in here, but it may not work for everyone. Again, it's what has worked for me, with much support. I really recommend getting support. Chapter six has many great concepts on the subject.

Why do we overeat? There are many reasons why we overeat. My husband can overeat on a holiday and be done with it. For me to do that would set up the bingeing cycle.

The recipes in this book work well for my plan of eating and may be adapted to yours. Friends have contributed too. They wanted to be a part of this story.

These recipes are all flour, sugar, and wheat free because that is what's worked for these friends and me.

Chapter Four
Why Do We Over Eat?

One of my coaching colleagues from Saudi Arabia said this profound thing; "Physical hunger comes gradually; emotional hunger bangs hard." Wow, is that ever true for me.

When I wake up in the morning, I'm hungry. And with good cause. I've been fasting anywhere from eight to twelve hours. I should be hungry in the morning. I always eat breakfast. Then as noon approaches, I begin to feel hungry again.

There are the times when I feel hungry between meals. When I follow my food plan, the meal I had previously was ample so there is not a physical reason for me to feel hungry. That means it's something else.

Somewhere as a young child, I got the notion that food takes away pain. I remember stealing candy out of my mom's underwear drawer when I was about four years old. I guess with six children, anything she really wanted for herself she had to hide. Candy she had to hide from me. When it came up missing, she used to blame my dad. There was no way I was going to admit I was into her stash. First of all, I thought that she would kill me. That's how my four-year-old mind worked. But more important, I did not want to lose my source of contraband.

I didn't realize it, but I pretty much blotted out unpleasant memories from my past. When I first gave up sugar after about a month, my long-term memory started to return. I sought counseling help to deal with that. This may not be true for everyone. But for me, my use of sugary foods began at a very early age and covered up some difficult moments in my life.

So eating for emotional reasons can be a big trigger. I did it so often, that I could no longer tell the difference between hunger and my emotions. When I felt uncomfortable, something went into my mouth. Over-eating became an abusive relationship for me. It would not leave me; I had to leave it, and needed help to do it.

Counseling really helped to sort out what was real hunger from emotional eating. Once I understood what was eating me, I didn't have to use food to take away feelings. Amazing, I did that so long, covered up feelings with food, that it was hard to tell them apart after a while.

Tired really feels like hunger. So does anxiety, fear, excitement, worry and sometimes happiness, anticipation, and love. Chapter six is entirely dedicated to emotional eating.

But there is hope. Feelings have a beginning and an end. If I can sit through them, they dissipate. And so does the hunger. Today I follow a set plan of eating which helps me to recognize that something is going on if I feel hunger in-between meals.

Most bouts of emotional hunger seem to stem from focusing on myself. If I'm having a pity-party, the best solution is to help someone else. It gives me great satisfaction to help others. Voilà. The feelings shift to happier moods.

Volunteer work is built into my schedule. It is sad that many people feel they don't have time to help others. When I was morbidly obese, I was focused only on myself. And food, of course. What I was going to eat? Where will I hide the wrappers? What time does that store close? Do they have what I want? How can I get away from people to have my binge? And on and on.

When I started taking an interest in others, I found that I was much less hungry in between meals. Little things keep my mood light too. It can be as small as not parking in the closest place to the grocery store. Oddly enough, it feels so good that overeating is the last thing that ventures into my mind.

As the parking space gift shows, helping others does not have to be big and dramatic. Some of the most fun I've had is to giving anonymously. For twelve days one year over the holidays, I'd went in to the office early, putting a gift on a different employee's desk every morning. It was fun to see them look forward to coming to work. Who would be the next person to get a gift? They tried to figure out who was doing it. One morning I left a gift on my own desk so I wouldn't get found out. It was a joyous holiday time for me. And I didn't overeat once.

I love going to the grocery stores over the holidays. Many of the stores have Christmas trees with paper ornaments that have names of underprivileged kids with a list of things they need or want. I usually pick a couple names to buy for. Because I was not blessed with children, I began doing this many years ago. Now I have three children and two grand kidlets by marriage. They give me plenty of opportunities to get out of self-centeredness.

So, look for places to get out of your self-centeredness. Maybe at your child's school or through your church. Maybe you have a neighbor who needs someone to visit for no reason. If you look, you'll find plenty of places to be generous with your time.

Because I've been blest with people giving me flowers over the years, there were an abundance of vases in my house. What fun it is to buy the inexpensive flowers at the grocery store and present them to a friend or co-worker in one of those vases. If you can get to the office early, before everyone else, leave a bouquet on a desk anonymously. What great fun and the perfect way to get out of my self centered-thinking.

Boredom is a one-way ticket to what I refer to as recreational eating. My suggestion to this is simple – get a life. There is no worldly excuse for boredom these days.

If you live in a community that has an association, see if there is a committee that needs your talent. Perhaps you have artistic talents hidden away. Take a class. Learn to paint. Write a book. Join a community theater or start a rock and roll band.

Join a gym. Read and write letters for the residents of a retirement home. Play checkers with your grandfather. Read to the students at the local elementary school. Tutor them in math and science. Sponsor a chess club. Have fun.

I bet that you can easily add to this list. If I focus on boredom, I'll be bored. If I focus on being an integral part of society, there won't be time to be bored. It's all a choice.

Since I retired from corporate America earlier this year, I frequently wonder when I had time to work. Writing this book has taken up hours of my time, as has my coaching practice. I'm going to school too. Can you imagine, fifty-seven years old and returning to academia? I love it.

Chapter Five
When It Is Not Physical Hunger

It could be emotional.

There are many triggers to picking up food when it's not physical. An hour after lunch, I should not be hungry. If I am following a good plan, it is easy to recognize that this is not physical hunger.

One of my client's tells this story of a day when he on a job out of town. He spent a long day working outside. It was a sticky-humid day, and he was looking forward to a nice meal, a hot shower, and a relaxing evening in his hotel room.

At the restaurant, he ordered dinner according to his food plan. It was an enjoyable meal, very satisfying. After dinner, however, there was an overwhelming sensation that he had to have something else. That quest took him to a Wendy's where he got a small frozen dessert and experienced the ah sensation.

During our session, we determined that he was tired. Tired felt like hungry. Now he has new information about himself. He knows that tired often feels like hungry and when tired, the appropriate action is to go to bed. Get some sleep.

One habit he had to break was the evening rattly bag syndrome. After dinner, he often consumed an entire bag of corn chips. Most likely, he was eating because he was bored, not because he was hungry. Now he rides a bike in the evenings after dinner, or he reads. But he doesn't eat.

Stress is another big trigger. A friend used to eat Reese's Peanut Butter Cups so fast, she wouldn't bother to remove the paper cups. This happened at work, in a high stress job. Sugar and fat. She had to find other ways of dealing with her stress rather than that candy.

That same friend had a secretary who totally got on my friend's nerves. When my friend changed her eating habits, she became disturbed that the secretary kept a jar of candy on her desk. My friend had a little pity party for herself. Didn't that secretary know that she was trying to lose weight? Of course, she didn't. And even if she did, she was not responsible for my friend's feelings. Not at all.

What a creative solution we came up with – every time the candy jar was the main focus, my friend gave her secretary a compliment. You might think that this is absurd but it worked. She no longer was upset by the candy jar, and they went on to become very good friends.

All of my previous diets failed because I felt deprived. I had to give up all those wonderful treats. Treats? I'd have a moment of ahhh and then I'd go right back to feeling deprived, resentful or angry. Diets made me feel deprived too. I couldn't have this or that. Poor me, poor me, pour me another bowl of cornflakes .

That deprivation mentality might have started in early childhood. I craved attention and did whatever I could to get it. Mom did the best she could but I was insatiable for her attention. When she couldn't devote special time to me, I comforted myself with food. Cornflakes was a big one. Any cereal, actually.

This feeling of deprivation followed me into adulthood. When a diet made me feel deprived, I was in big trouble. It would only be a matter of time before a binge made that diet history. The deprivation mentality only changed when I saw that overeating – because it kept me from living – was the true deprivation, not doing without certain foods.

I don't feel that way today. I gave up so much of life to support my eating habit. Morbid obesity made many activities impossible. Plus, I deprived myself of good health.

Today I make doggone sure that my meals are attractive, tasty, and satisfying. I really enjoy my meals and don't miss the trigger foods. Yes, you can look forward to attractive, tasty and satisfying meals too. It is critical, in my estimation, to watch out for that feeling of deprivation. It has been my catalyst to a binge.

Fear is a great motivator for overeating. In 2004, my husband David and I were living in Orlando where we experienced three hurricanes over a two month period. The first one, Charley, was fast and furious. I had often heard people describing that freight train going by, and we heard that. I was terrified. The wind actually pulled our French doors outward. Later we learned that a tornado went directly over our house, taking out much of the roof shingles, the back fence, and several trees.

In the midst of this, I asked Dave if he wanted a snack. He looked at me as if I had grown two heads.

"No."

Then he realized I was scared, petrified really, and sat with me on the couch. I'll tell you what, terror sure felt hungry that night.

Anger is another real trigger for me. It used to be very difficult for me to express anger appropriately. I would either rip somebody's head off or hide in a corner having my very own little pity party. I ate at the anger. It takes a lot of food to dispel anger and in the end, I had a stomach ache and the anger. Being angry at someone and eating over it is like me taking poison and expecting the other person to die.

Once in high school, I was angry with a girl-friend who was flirting with my boyfriend. I'd fix her: I recall eating a whole jar of hot peppers and paying dearly for several days with major pain in the tummy. I can't even remember what happened with the boyfriend, but I still remember how awful I felt after eating all those peppers.

Confusion, vulnerability, sadness, resentment, grief, embarrassment, disappointment-- you can add to that list, I am sure. It took a long time to sort out genuine feelings from hunger. Sometimes positive feelings are more confusing than the negative ones.

Love often feels like hunger. As a child after school, my mother would be waiting with milk and cookies. She loved me. I cherished that time with her without my brothers and sisters.

For our birthday, she always cooked our favorite meals. That really meant that she loved me. I was allowed to pick the entire menu, which was always a big combination of grease and flour, followed by some sugary concoction for dessert.

As a young bride, I cooked great meals for my new husband. That meant I loved him. And if he ate my meals, he loved me. If he really raved about my cooking, he really loved me. More cause for hunger and love getting mixed up in my head and feeling the same.

Have you ever celebrated with food? We sure did at my house growing up. The hub of activity in our home was the kitchen. Birthdays, weddings, anniversaries, promotions, or visiting relatives were all excuses for food fests.

My Uncle John would come to visit from Baltimore, and he brought those yummy Maryland crabs. Our table would be covered with newspapers as we sat down for hours talking, laughing, and eating with Uncle John. What a fond memory.

So many of my childhood memories are associated with food. As Catholics, we did not eat meat on Fridays but it never felt like a hardship to me. My mother made home made potato soup, grilled cheese sandwiches, and her special apple dumplings. She fixed love in the kitchen.

Sunday mornings was when we got some of Dad's kitchen lovin'. He cooked breakfast after church. Poached eggs and bacon, or sometimes he'd scramble eggs with onions and bacon. Dad really loved us because he cooked great breakfast on Sunday.

You can see where I developed strong ties to food and feelings. What a mess it was to straighten that all out. It all boils down to doing the work of sorting out the feelings and learning how to express them appropriately. Food will not make feelings dissipate. Dealing with the situation that causes the feelings will.

Here you may need professional help from a counselor, minister, or coach to sort this stuff out. Get the help you need to learn the difference between feelings and hunger. Don't resent the money – remember all the money you put into getting your drug of choice – food.

I believe my long-term memory was also affected by sugar. I blotted out some painful memories with candy, cookies, and junk food. I stopped eating sweets in May of 1993 and a flood of memories came, along with the feelings that accompanied them. Here therapy was quite helpful, to get all that straightened out in my head. It was worth the financial investment in myself to get that emotional help. Permanent weight loss was only possible when I didn't need to eat at my feelings.

Feelings are not facts, you know. If you've ignored them for any period of time, when they come back, they seem so much more intense. I had huge emotional swings after coming out from my sugar-fogged years. When I started to experience anger, at first it was rage. I was wildly excited or deeply depressed.

Gradually, I learned how to feel a feeling and move on. It did not have to consume me, take over my life. Then I didn't have to eat over them. I learned new coping skills to deal with life on life's terms and not use food as a drug to stuff the emotions down. Today, I'm much more in the middle of the road when it comes to emotions.

Swinging forward, today I savor feelings. When my little granddaughter gives me a big, juicy hug, I get a beautiful rush of emotions. It is delicious. Man, what I was missing for the sake of food.

Apprehension was all but eliminated when I was face first in a pizza. Apprehension could be a first line signal that perhaps some greater action is required. If I don't feel it, I cannot react to it. I can react appropriately today when apprehensive.

Now that I am living a full-feeling life, I wonder why I thought life was so bad that I had to zone out the way I did. It wasn't so bad. It was pretty good when you get right down to it. Sure, bad things happen to good people, and we all find our ways to survive that stuff. I used food. It was a drug that I could get to as a young child and kept using well into my adulthood.

At some point, however, it became a way of life. Feeling was food. One meant the other. It took a long time to break that association. I needed help.

If you suspect that you might be using food to cover up feelings, please, please, get some help. Your health insurance may cover counseling. There are eating disorder counselors who deal with this sort of thing and can help you to get down to what is eating you. Speak to your minister, rabbi, priest at church or your family doctor. A full life is worth it. You can loosen the grip that food has on you.

Chapter Six
Get Support

Do you think that any team can win a football game if the only player on the field was the quarterback? Even if he was the greatest quarterback in history, by himself, he cannot win the game. There must be other players to catch the ball and protect the quarterback. It is necessary to block the other team from scoring.

This analogy made great sense to me. My diets were a lonely venture. Even some of the diet clubs where we'd go weigh in and sit through a class on what to do to stay on our diets. I'd go there and smile at people, but I didn't connect with anyone.

When it came to losing weight, I was on my own. Worse, when they weighed me, if the number went up from the week before, I felt humiliated. I couldn't wait to get out of there.

So, playing together makes a great football team. Could that work with my new philosophies on food and weight loss? Finding the right support can be very challenging.

My family was always there for me but it turned out that family was not the best support. Food is love in most families. You know their lines:

"One bite won't hurt."

"I made this just for you."

"Are you going to be on that diet forever?"

"All you need is a little willpower."

Well, if willpower was all I needed, the first diet I went on at age sixteen would have worked, and I'd never have gained over one hundred pounds. Most of my family really does have willpower. So do I, for that matter. They don't understand why willpower didn't work for me with regard to dieting. I don't even really know why my willpower didn't work on diets. It did in many areas of my life, but not where food was concerned.

Plus, I lost credibility with my family. Whenever I went on a new diet, I'd become the expert. All I'd talk about was my latest harebrained dieting adventure. They'd bide their time and sooner or later, I'd be the heavy sister. Again.

"Oh Gerri, you have such a pretty face." How I hated to hear that line. Just keep that in mind, family may not be the best support. So, where can you go to get help?

The very best support I've seen is the twelve step programs, fashioned after Alcoholics Anonymous. Overeaters Anonymous has a website, www.oa.org. There you can find local, telephone and online meetings, as well as support.

There are other twelve step fellowships just for food: Food Addicts Anonymous, Compulsive Eaters Anonymous, Anorexic/Bulimics Anonymous, Recovering Food Addicts. At last count I heard there were twenty-seven different twelve step groups for food abuse.

One reason that you need support is identifying trigger foods. Then when giving up trigger foods there are sometimes withdrawal symptoms that others can help you identify and manage. And then there are the feelings and memories that come up once the food is gone.

Sugar was the first thing I discovered that set up cravings, and I gave it up entirely. At first I stopped eating what I call recreational sugar: cookies, cakes, candy, high sugar snacks.

I suffered what some would refer to as withdrawal symptoms. My body ached. I had a terrible headache and didn't sleep well. Looking back, it was not fun. I don't think I'll ever start eating sugar products again. I never want to go through the withdrawal discomfort again.

After about four weeks, I started remembering some things from childhood that were quite distressing. I sought counseling and received a great deal of support in group therapy. In fact, from late 1993 until early 1998, I lived in a halfway house setting, with other people who also went to counseling for our eating disorders.

I never regretted that, as I learned how to lean on others for support during this time. I also learned to cook and shop as well as how to say, "No, thank you," when offered the foods I no longer ate. It was a support group that I could count on when I needed help.

Many churches have support groups that offer a spiritual approach to eating. Check with your church to see if they offer anything that may be helpful to you or if one can be started.

Some gyms also can be quite supportive. Curves, the chain that caters to women, takes a holistic approach with their clients to help them lose weight in a healthy way and keep it off through proper nutrition and exercise. At the larger gyms, I've made good friends with people in the aerobics classes. We all have a common purpose, to lose weight and keep it off.

You might even have a close group of friends who'd hold you accountable. The support of friendship was paramount for me in not only losing weight, but also in maintaining a healthy body size. Even after fourteen years, I still have and need a strong support system.

Some of the weight loss programs offer support in the form of weekly meetings. Unfortunately for me, I'd go to the meetings, weigh in, leave, binge for a few days, and then starve until the next weigh in. For me to succeed, more accountability was needed between the weekly meetings.

You may also want to hire a life/health coach, who'll help you develop a mindful eating plan that works for you. I am coaching people now, who are making remarkable changes in their lives to achieve permanent weight loss. A good coach will support you to find the right food and exercise plan that works for you, not a cookie-cutter plan. A good coach has no ulterior motives and will work with you to succeed.

There is no right or wrong support. Pick what feels right and if what you select at first does not work, try another. Don't give up. I struggled with diets and weight loss schemes until I was forty-three before finding the right combination.

I still occasionally get thoughts to eat off my plan. My head will present very credible scenarios. It is almost comical how often my thoughts will seem so logical that food could solve a problem.

I look at it this way; I spent forty-three years dealing with my life with food as a solution. It worked, or so it seemed to work. My mind would be off the problem and on to getting the food. Naturally, with all that experience, it's understandable that my brain would think of using food to deal with feelings.

So, I've learned to say, "Thank you for sharing," to myself. The second time, I'll kind of warn myself. "Look, if you continue with this line of thinking, I'll have to tell on you. Cookies do not solve problems." The third time, I'll call a friend and tell on myself.

"You won't believe how I'm thinking. I have something going on and I'm thinking that a cookie is going to solve the problem." My friends now are used to me doing this and laugh about it with me. The amazing thing is that after this three step process, the thought to eat my way through any situation goes away. Putting a voice to the insanity of it all helps dissipate the food thoughts.

So, build a circle of support for yourself. If one doesn't work, try again until you find something that does work. Don't give up. For me, this is a critical part of my success.

To recap, some ideas for getting help are:
> Church
> Coaching
> Friends
> Gym
> Therapy
> Twelve Step groups such as
>> Overeaters Anonymous
> Weight-loss groups

Chapter Seven
Coaching For Support

It is amazing; once my food problem became manageable, how much more there was for me in life. One way I've found for getting the most out of my whole life, is through the help of a life coach. Using a life/health coach is a great way to not only find support for your weight loss, but also to build a bridge from where you are now to where you want to be with other areas of your life. You can change from your current eating habits to a healthier way of life with permanent weight loss.

We each have the solution in us but sometimes it's hard to see because we're overwhelmed or so far down in our rut, we can't see over the sides. A good coach will help you find what works for you. Some of us need a plan that is tailored to us. The perfect solution is inside you. What you need is someone to coach it out of you.

As a life/health coach, I partner with people who in the past, have not enjoyed the success of maintaining weight loss. No, I am not a health care professional. I am not a nutritionist. What I am is someone who not only has lost over one hundred pounds, but also has kept it off for over fourteen years. And who is helping my clients develop a strategy that works for them.

In our coaching sessions, we look at the role food plays in the client's life and how it impacts health, appearance, social life, career – all aspects of life. Each of these things may be affected by an unhealthy relationship with food. We look at the present, what is going on right now.

Next, through thoughtful questioning, we determine where the client would like to be at a specific point in the future. Then we have fun. We build a bridge from where they are, to where they want to be. It's an individualized, unique plan to reach their specific health and weight loss goals. When the client creates the goal, he or she is more likely to achieve it.

We often find that the client is engaged in mindless eating. Our journey is to change mindless to mindful eating. What a privilege to work with clients who really want to change their lives. I know what it is like to feel hopeless, like I could never lose weight and keep it off. If you have also felt this way, a coach may be just the answer for you.

I am excited to share my ideas with clients. I am excited to help you determine what works for you and what does not. So what if you've failed in the past? So have I. That can change, if you want it to change, if you really, really want it.

Once the food starts to take it's rightful place, the roller coaster of life takes off. Wahoo! Really, life will take on a whole new meaning. I am watching clients who have put dreams on a back burner ignite that fire again. Some return to college. One in her fifties is learning to ride a Harley motorcycle. Another is on her way to becoming a doctor.

There is life after food.

What's your dream? What's stopping you? Why haven't diets worked for you? Perhaps you are experiencing success in other areas of your life -- work, marriage, raising a family, in social settings, but when it comes to food something is missing.

With a coach, in addition to looking at what you're eating, you can look at what's eating you. This may be the first time you've considered what might be a factor in your overeating. Perhaps there are button-pushing areas of your life that set up bingeing.

Not a binger? Okay, maybe you did more grazing, which is another of my old habits. I couldn't understand why I was so fat, after all, I ate like a bird. The trouble, someone told me, is that birds, over the course of a day, eat two and a half times their body weight. I was consuming double what my body required, since I was nearly double a normal body size.

This is a fact. In order to gain weight, we must eat more than our body requires. And in order to become morbidly obese as I was, we must eat much more than our body requires. Whether bingeing or grazing, calories in excess of what we need will result in weight gain.

Perhaps you are not obese or even over-weight. Perhaps you are just a few pounds overweight. Many overeat but control it with incessant calorie counting, exercising, or purging through vomiting or laxatives. Overeating doesn't start on a spoon or in a rattly bag, it starts between our ears.

Normal physical hunger comes gradually. Emotional hunger often bangs on the door, barges right in, and immediately consumes the thinking process until sated with food. Salty, sweet, crunchy, creamy -- each of us may have a different fix, but like the cocaine addict, when that door banging starts, it will not subside until satisfied with the drug of choice, whether it's food or something else.

As I've said, when I eat certain foods, I crave more. Identifying these foods has been paramount to my losing and maintaining a permanent weight loss. My clients are los-ing weight. Why? Because they are crafting plans and strategies to develop better eat-ing habits.

There are often emotional upheavals that contribute to overeating. Even if you deal with trigger foods, if you don't identify and modify overeating behaviors, you probably will return to overeating.

Therapy is a great way to discover why we developed those coping mechanisms. If you think you need some counseling, try it. You are worth it. In coaching, we start with the present and work toward putting any messes behind us, pick up the pieces and move in a positive, forward direction. Coaching and counseling can work for you.

Whether or not you know why you started eating the way you do doesn't matter in coaching. Replacing the poor eating behaviors with healthy eating behaviors is what's important in my practice.

Since I'm not a victim of food abuse any more, my coach and I were able to look immediately at other areas of my life where I wanted to excel. Without the fog of excess food, I am clear and available to think about what I want to do, where I want to go, what great goals I want to accomplish in my life.

When the overeating finally ended, I found that I had an immense amount of time on my hands. The last fourteen years have been amazing for me. Before I dreamed, but slowly and methodically, the dreams went away, replaced by constant eating. Soon, all that was left for me was my friend food.

But not now. My dreams are coming true. For many years, I was so driven by food, that I could not think my way out of a wet paper bag. Now I'm clear and set out to pursue a dream I'd had since childhood – writing a book. I wrote a book. This book.

My coach held me accountable, week after week and slowly but surely, the book came out of my head and onto the computer. Do you have dreams like this too? Why not consider coaching to make them come true for you?

Not only that, I walked away from a twenty-five year career where I was safe. I had a good job, making decent money. Today, I am coaching and loving every minute of it. I don't have to play it safe, I can take a risk.

I wonder what fantastic things lie ahead for you? Once food no longer has you in its grip and you are choosing to work with a coach, the only limit is your imagination. As a coach, my only motive is the success of my clients. I partner with clients who want to succeed in taking off those unwanted pounds, change their life, and reach goals they never dreamed possible.

If you want to know more about coaching there is a great deal of information on the internet. One is the International Federation of Coaches site, http://www.coachfederation.org/ICF/. There is information on how to find a coach.

You can also visit the Coach-U website for a list of credentialed coaches, http://www.coachinc.com/CoachU/. Currently, the industry is not regulated, but Coach-U offer education for credentials in this field.

Most coaches will extend a complimentary first session so that you can see if their style works for you. Prior to that first session, I e-mail a few thought provoking questions. My clients are already intrigued about how to achieve their goals. I coach most of my clients by telephone. I live in Florida and some clients are as far away as California.

Whether you are dealing with maintaining healthy weight or other challenges, you can add value to your life with a coach. Health, personal and business coaching is an ongoing professional relationship that helps people produce extraordinary results with many areas of their life. Learn how it works and how it can add value to your life. Why shouldn't you have a coach too?

Chapter Eight
Trust God and Buy Broccoli

Oh boy, here comes the God thing. Hang in there. It does not matter if you are a churchgoer or not, this isn't about bible-thumping. This is about permanent weight loss. It took a long time for me to be open to understand what I could not find with diet, exercise, and weight-loss schemes alone.

I grew up in a Christian family, and our religious tradition included church on Sunday. I went to a Christian school, from kindergarten through high school graduation. And I ended up fat.

As I gained weight in adulthood, I prayed that God would make me thin. But He didn't. I had a very warped vision of God. He was somewhere in-between Santa Claus and a jail executioner. Prayer wasn't going to magically make me thin. Eating in a manner to lose weight did.

By the time I was willing to consider God as part of the solution, food had become my higher power. It was a power in my life to be sure. Every time I vowed in the morning to go on a diet, and then broke that diet by noon, food reinforced itself as my god.

I had a spiritual experience in 1993 that lead me to see where God could indeed be there for me, where food was concerned. Seeing that my best thinking brought me to near suicide was the bottom I needed. It was life changing.

It's not really about broccoli you know. It's about taking action. If I have a candy bar an inch from my mouth, and I say, "God, please help me to not eat this candy bar," odds are pretty good I won't be getting a lightning bolt from heaven saying, "Stop." At that stage, I don't really want His help. I want that candy bar. I've made a decision to make that candy bar a god. I have no alternatives at that moment to do anything other than eat that candy bar.

And another.

And another.

And another.

One candy bar leads to a dozen for me.

Now, I pray every morning, asking God to help me make good decisions about my food. I write what I am going to eat that day in my food journal. I try not to change it. Of course, life happens. If we get a last minute dinner invitation, I'll order one of my restaurant standbys.

Each evening, I'm back down on my knees in gratitude for another day of sane, healthy eating. I know in my heart that somebody or something is helping me. Otherwise, the first diet I ever went on would have worked. While I exhibit fairly good willpower in many areas of my life, it was not much help when it came to food.

Even now I am much better at overeating than I am at mindful eating. Why? At age forty-three, when life as I knew it changed, I had accumulated sixteen thousand days in my over-eating lifestyle. As of mid-2007, I have over five thousand days of this new lifestyle. Which do you think I am better at? The old eating habits, by sheer repetition, are more ingrained in me than this new way of life.

So, if God can help me change that, I'm grabbing on. Let's face it, the diets didn't work for me. If they did, I'd be a lifetime member of Weight Watchers. I am not; I was not after several tries at Weight Watchers. I needed something different.

I have a great core of support today. My friends all know how I eat and they are there for me. When that refrigerator starts calling me (and it does at times), I can call a friend, just to talk. Those friends? They're God with skin. They become stronger for me than the food that is singing in the refrigerator.

I found something spiritual about staying on my food plan. My mind is free to think about other things. I plan my food, prepare it, weigh and/or measure it, and eat it. Then I don't have to think about it any more until time for the next meal. I have time to think about other worthwhile things in my life. I had no idea how much thinking time was wasted when I dedicated it to food and the pursuit of food.

I feel so much peace and serenity today, now that I have learned to ask God for help. Do you know that I asked for His help when I was thinking of having a good man in my life? A friend suggested that I write a letter to God and tell Him what I wanted in a man.

"Why, that's the craziest thing I've ever heard of," I said to my friend. Yeah? She reminded me that every day I start out on my knees and ask God to help me with my food and every night I am back down there, thanking Him for the help that day.

So if God could help me with the biggest hurdle in my life, that of food, why couldn't He also help me with something as important as a relationship? So, I wrote the letter.

My friend advised me to be very specific. If money or looks were important, write it down. If religious convictions or lack of that was important, write it down. It took me several days of thinking and praying before the letter was complete. Or at least I thought it was complete.

During this process of composing the letter, a well-intentioned friend called, wanting to fix me up on a blind date with an engineer. As I waited at the restaurant, I wondered if this was the answer to the letter, although I had not yet actually sent it to God. As my date walked up, wearing what he described on the phone, I smiled and he smiled back.

To my horror, his teeth were terrible. They were obviously not well cared for. I thought, if he cannot take care of his teeth, how can he take care of me? And there was no way I was going to kiss him. The date was pleasant enough, but I knew he was not my knight in shining armor. I went home and added "good dental hygiene" to my list of qualifications for that special man for God to send me.

About a week later, I thought the letter was complete so I got down on my knees and read it to God. How long would He take? Would He say, "Okay," and send this man to me?

This perfect man had to be a widower, not divorced (because it seemed to me divorced men were really only interested in women who were for sale for the price of dinner. Since I never had children of my own, I hoped he would have grown children and they'd like me. Grandchildren would be nice too. This guy would enjoy sports because I scuba dive and enjoy NASCAR. He would like to go to amusement parks. I lived very near to Disney. I had hoped he'd be my religion, a non-drinker, non-smoker, and able to support himself financially. There was more but that was the gist of it. Oh, yes, and good dental hygiene.

A few days later, a friend sent me this hug in an e-mail. I had to click on the hug and it sent me to the website AOL's Love Connection. What in the world? I finally figured out what it was and thought, this is like a boyfriend grocery store. I'm not that desperate. God wouldn't be sending me here. I closed the website.

A few days later, I peeked at it again. And, there was this man, who was everything I had written in the letter. Amazing. A little moment of panic however, as he was looking for a woman five-foot, seven-inches tall or taller. In my highest pair of stiletto heels, I'd not clear five feet, six inches, but I hoped maybe the height would not be too great a factor.

I took a chance and e-mailed him. Turns out, the tall thing was just a guy being a guy – his former wife was that tall and he had no point of reference other than that when he placed his ad. He didn't mind at all that I was only five-feet, three-inches tall.

We started e-mailing back and forth, graduated to telephone calls, and finally went for a first date. I was smitten and so was he.

We dated for a year, got engaged, and married the following year in 2001. I never imagined being in such a wonderful, rewarding relationship. I truly believed God would help me with finding the right man, and He did.

And I truly believe that God -- the Universe, Power, or whatever you want to call it/him/her — wants more for me than I could ever want for myself. He wants abundance for me.

I do have a choice today though. Where do I want that abundance? Do I want it in my life, or do I want it in my mouth. I've experienced both today and much prefer His Abundance in my life.

Chapter Nine
Thank You For Sharing

Let's see. How many years did I solve problems with food? Given that I can remember sneaking food at age four, it was probably close to forty. I became quite good at using food to deal with emotional issues. The problems never really went away, and then there were two problem -- the one that I ate over and then the remorse from having over eaten.

I sometimes would joke and say that if the house caught on fire, I'd go buy a box of cream-filled donuts before I'd dial 9-1-1. That's pretty scary. There was some truth to this. If I experienced any kind of fear, anxiety, or excitement, it felt like hunger. I turned to food for comfort. It must have worked once in early childhood, and then I sought that same feeling for the next forty years. Even though it did not fix problems, I kept turning to food anyway. It was the only thing I knew.

My head got very used to this pattern, just as Pavlov's dogs salivated at the sound of a bell, I turned to food as soon as any emotion spiked. It would numb me out for a bit, but it took more and more food to get to that ahhhh moment. I tried many combinations too, -- salty and crunchy or soft and creamy.

I imagine that food was some sort of coping thing for me and thank God it worked at times. Maybe I'd have gone right out of my mind if I couldn't have taken the edge off of some of those feelings. Eventually, after repeating this over and over (get a feeling, put something in my mouth), it became almost reflex. Soon feelings felt like ... hungry.

As a result, I no longer really had true feelings. And not only did I dilute the yucky ones, inadvertently, I dulled the good ones, too. I rarely felt exuberance, deep happiness, or love. Only hungry.

I also developed some hand-to-mouth habits too. Early in my transition to good eating habits, I had cooked a turkey and was packaging it into three or four ounce servings for the freezer, a convenient way to grab meals with my hectic schedule.

But my fingers had a mind of their own. I'd slice the turkey and my fingers would naturally gravitate to my mouth. It was very frustrating. My then-husband was in the other room and I asked him to come out and keep me company so I wouldn't mindlessly pop pieces of turkey into my mouth.

He stood behind me and with each swipe of the knife, up would go my hand and he'd push it back down. It became comical. Hysterically funny. We laughed so hard there were tears in both our eyes. We finally switched places, and he carved the turkey while I watched. I just couldn't do it by myself. I needed help. My hand was so used to going to my mouth that it just naturally went there.

How was I going to break such a strong reflex? It takes a long time to make new habits. It made me a little crazy in the beginning.

For the first five years of my new eating habits, I stopped watching television because it was a huge trigger for me. I vegged out in front of the boob tube, eating until I could not move off the couch. The association was very strong.

Today I can occasionally eat with Dave in the living room, in front of the television. My present life feels so much better that I finally want it more than the feeling that I got from bingeing.

My old thinking can return in a heartbeat, from out of nowhere. I was in my new life about three years and things were going fairly well. I lived in beautiful downtown Winter Park, right on Lake Osceola. I was walking back from the post office on a picture perfect day. The sun was shining. The birds singing in the trees. I was out in the fresh air.

I had a good job, amazing friends, and thought, "It doesn't get much better than this." The next thing I thought was, "You can stop and get a nice ice cream cone." Woah, where'd that come from?

I had finished lunch about an hour earlier. I was not hungry, and it was a perfect day. But it wasn't enough. My old thought pattern was to make it even better with food. I wasn't tired, bored, or lonely, and I never, never ate one ice cream cone. I knew where that would lead — to gallons of ice cream and morbid obesity.

So, I said to myself, "Thank you for sharing." Ha. That was funny. But it was true.

Did you ever smoke? I did. And years after I quit, sometimes I'd reach into my purse for a cigarette and it would hit me that I hadn't had a cigarette in forever. Why is that? Reinforced behavior. And so it was with the food, a very reinforced habit.

I just figure that when I am forty-three years on this side of good eating, reaching for food will not be a reflex action as it was in my first forty-three years. Or a cigarette.

So today, when I get a thought that something to eat would solve a problem, I thank my head for sharing. And I don't eat. No matter what. If I am hungry in-between meals, it is not physical hunger.

This is where a set food plan is so invaluable. If meals are balanced and they have a beginning and an end, it is easy to recognize that an hour after a meal, if I feel hungry, it's not for food.

I like to write down my plan for the day either the night before, or at least that morning. It really helps during those times when I get hungry in-between meals. I know what and when I should eat my next meal. Sometimes I do need to change it, because I live life on life's terms, and not necessarily on a food plan's terms. It really helps me to have a plan to follow.

Calling friends has been a great alternative to snacking.When David and I were planning our wedding, it seemed I was hungry all the time. Often late at night I'd be stark-raving starving. At least it felt that way. Most local friends were already in bed, but I had a friend in California who was three hours behind me.

I'd call Lynda, and we had this standing joke. I'd say, "It's the Bride." I'd tell her I was starving, and then she'd let me talk. After a bit, I could process what was really going on for me. I'd know what was underneath the hunger. It was worry about the wedding plans, wondering if we had invited enough people, or too many, to the reception.

When it wasn't anxiety, it was just plain old stupid in love with that handsome man. I was so happy to be marrying him. Those were new feelings. I never really felt deep happiness like this because I shoved food in my mouth when the slightest indication of a feeling surfaced.

"Thank you for sharing." Yeah, that works pretty good.

Chapter 9

Chapter Ten
One Bite Won't Hurt

They just don't get it. One bite does hurt somebody like me. But they just don't get it.

My younger brother Tom keeps himself in pretty good shape. For that matter, all my five brothers and sisters look good. None of them became morbidly obese like me. Tom says all I need is willpower. That may work for Tom, but it doesn't work for me so I just stopped trying to explain. He doesn't get it. He'll never get it.

The point here is that if I don't eat a bite of cake, I cannot eat the whole cake. Maybe you can eat a bite of cake and stop, but I just can't. And even if through some miracle I do have only that one bite, the mental torture that follows is unbearable.

My mind is relentless. I'll spend hours rationalizing, making deals with myself, talking myself into more, out of more ad nausea. No thank you. It is easier to just not eat that first bite.

And food is love in my family. "Here, I made this just for you." Ever heard that one before? Ah, yes, turn it down and you may as well slap 'em in the face.

The kitchen was the hub of love in our home. What a small kitchen it was too. How my mother ever crammed eight of us in there, I'll never know.

On our birthdays, we'd get whatever meal we wanted. Mom loved us real good with her cooking. Even today, there are special desserts that she makes that taste like love.

How do you deal with this? It's hard. "No thank you." Just doesn't cut it. I've had to learn how to gently turn down food without saying, "I don't want your love, Mom." That's real hard.

I had to develop techniques to stay on my plan around family and not appear to be turning down their love offerings.

This has worked – when someone walks up with a goodie, thank them and take the plate. Just set the plate down on a table. Wait a few minutes, and then walk away. Go to another area of the room. People leave food on tables all the time. They forgot about it. I've watched them do it. If the person giving the goodie is persistent, try telling them that you've just eaten not too long ago and want to save it for later. That has worked for me too.

At parties, I've already just said, "No, thank you, I'm full," or "I just couldn't eat another bite." Sometimes that works. However, some people are persistent and don't take no for an answer.

If there is enough protest, I've occasionally said that I have food allergies. That usually does it, but once someone asked me what would happen if I ate it. I said, "I swell up real bad." That's true. Two hundred and fifty pounds is extremely swollen, and that is where a bite of some foods will ultimately take me.

On occasion, I've even told people that I don't like chocolate or some other obvious ingredient. Most of the time that works.

Some people will go into a big story about another person they know who doesn't like chocolate. Be polite, listen to their story but most more important, stick to your guns, and don't take that first bite, no matter what.

You can also ask your host to wrap it up for later. If you can take it home without eating it yourself, take it home for your family. If I am going to do that, I'll put it in the trunk so I'm not tempted to eat it in the car. Maybe you need to do that too. Or don't take it if there is any chance that you might eat it. Just drop it in a trash can.

Waste it? Oh, no, what would your mother say about wasting food? What about all those kids in China who'll go hungry tonight?

Here's the bottom line -- wasted food is wasted food. Whether you throw it in the trash or put it in your body, it's wasted. If it is food that sets up bingeing, better throw it in the trash. If it is food that surpasses the calories you need in a day for weight gain or loss, it is trash. If you've already had your meals for the day, and you eat it, you are treating your body like a trash can.

Food is not love, even if it feels like love. Food is food. And one bite will hurt. You never have to eat for somebody else again. Isn't that a relief?

"No," is a complete sentence. I've occasionally just said no. And when I've turned down food, the presenter can sometimes follow it with a question, like, "Why not?" Today I know that I'm not required to answer questions. Sometimes I answer a question with another question, like, "Why do you ask?"

These actions are not going to feel natural at first. When I first started taking care of myself, I was like a verbal bull in a china cabinet. We were celebrating something at my sister Joanne's house in Pennsylvania. I had flown up for the occasion and hadn't seen my family for a few years.

They were all so happy that I had lost my weight and seemed to be doing so well on my new diet. Hey, let them call it whatever they want to. My dad, what a sweetie pie, walked up to me with a plate of cold shrimp and cocktail sauce. He said the dreaded, "Here Gerri, I made this just for you."

Well, out came my blame thrower, and I verbally blasted that sweet man from here to hell and back: "Dad, I told you I'm not eating in between meals" I watched his face just sink in disappointment. I had under-developed coping skills on how to treat people who were well intentioned and trying to demonstrate their love and caring for me.

What to do, what to do? How could I turn this around? I prayed and asked God for some help. Then I had this wonderful inspiration. I walked over to my dad and hugged him. I said, "Dad, it was so thoughtful of you to make a special treat for me. I know how much you love me. Would it be okay with you if I have that shrimp with my dinner later? I'm really trying not to eat in between meals."

As I talked, I watched his dejected demeanor change. His eyes took on their previous sparkle, and he reveled in the moment that his love offering was received. It worked.

In the initial dealings with family and friends, as we train them on how we need to be treated with our new eating patterns, we probably will make some mistakes and create hurt feelings. It gets better, trust me. Just remember, one bite will hurt. Don't eat it, no matter what.

Chapter Eleven
Eating In Restaurants

Oh boy, my old binge stomping grounds – restaurants. I had to learn all new coping skills. Today I can eat anywhere – fast food, Chinese, Italian, Greek. In fourteen years, I have not found a restaurant where I could not get a meal that conforms to this great plan I follow. I can stay on my plan anywhere, and I can be spontaneous too.

Buffets, too? Yup.

How can that be? First line of defense at buffets is only one trip. Put what appears to be a normal portion of protein, vegetables, starch, and salad on your plate. No seconds.

To judge protein, take two pieces of chicken, baked not fried or breaded. Sometimes

I actually weigh the meat from the buffet. I purchased a small purse-sized scale on the internet. At buffets, I do weigh my portions of protein more than I don't as I don't have a good point of reference on how much I'm eating. Some say you can take a portion the size of your fist or of a deck of cards.

That doesn't work so good for me. My inventive little mind has a warped idea of how big my fist is and likes big card decks. So I weigh it. The first time I did this, I felt very awkward and conspicuous but it turned out that it wasn't a big deal. No one said a word about it. Believe it or not people aren't paying attention to me in restaurants. They are engrossed in their own meals, their own plates, their own family and friends, and could care less if I am weighing my food.

However, sometimes my head wants me to believe it's a big deal. That thank-you-for-sharing message works here as well.

If I get a baked potato, I only eat half of it or weigh it to four ounces. I don't weigh vegetables in restaurants as I cannot ever remember bingeing on carrots or green beans.

And certainly not broccoli. If you have, you might consider weighing them.

Also if there is fresh fruit and that is on your plan, have a piece of that too. Watch for fruits salads as they often are made with sugar. I avoid them.

Hidden sugars and fats are the real problem in restaurants. Buffet green beans often have bacon in them. Safe salad dressings for me include ranch, blue cheese, or good old oil and vinegar. Carrots are often sugared too. Vegetables are sometimes loaded down with butter. Fats and sugar are how restaurants make their food taste so good. But you can do it. You can eat in a restaurant in a sane, mindful way.

When I have occasion to stop at a fast food restaurant, I have some favorites. First on my list is Subway. You've probably seen their commercials featuring Jared Fogel. He's the guy who lost almost two hundred-fifty pounds by just eating Subway sandwiches. They also have an excellent variety of salads. The Fresh Fit menu provides healthy choices for family and friends.

Wendy's has several salads that work, as well as their chili and a baked potato. However, sometimes one potato at Wendy's could feed a family of four. If you are served one of those giant potatoes, weigh it or eat only a third. Be mindful.

You can also get a Tendergrill Garden Salad at Burger King. It has plenty of greens with chicken. McDonald's has both a Caesar Salad with Grilled Chicken and an Asian Salad with Grilled Chicken that will work. I have weighed the protein at home and it comes up short, but there is also cheese on most of their salads.

Most of the fast food restaurants have web pages. If there is one you really like, go to their website and see what they have which works for your plan.

Eating at diners can work too. While you can get more than enough calories for a week with one Grand Slam breakfast at Denny's, you can order a reasonable and sane meal there too. Grilled chicken, steak, fish, baked potato, salad, tomato slices all these items can be used to add up to a lunch or dinner that works with a plan of eating for weight loss or maintenance. A veggie omelette is a great protein, not only for breakfast, but also lunch or dinner. Skip the hash browns, way too much fat. Grits make an okay grain, but be aware of the hidden, or not so hidden, butter.

Even at an Italian restaurant such as Olive Garden or Macaroni Grill, you can stick to your eating plan. They have many dishes which do not include pasta. Before you go, check their website for chicken and fish dishes that include vegetables, rice or potatoes, and salads.

I do have a little problem with the head chatter in restaurants where they put stuff on the table to munch on before the food comes. Roadhouse Grill features a big bucket of peanuts. Mexican restaurants have the chips and salsa. In Chinese restaurants, they give you those little fried noodles. You do not have to eat these things.

When with my husband, I'll just remind him that I don't eat nuts or chips or Chinese noodles. That quiets down the head chatter -- that rationalization I have a tendency to start up. If I tell on myself to my husband that chatter usually goes away immediately. Once again, if I don't eat one peanut, I won't have to worry about eating the entire bucket, right?

Waiters don't mind helping, I've learned. When I approach my server asking for help, and not as another bimbo on a diet, I am well taken care of. But you have to ask questions. Keeping it simple is very effective. I have told waiters that I am allergic to sugar and flour, so they checked the order with the chef. Sometimes the chef will even come out to speak with me.

I know what I want before I got to most restaurants. I don't menu surf. You can ask for chicken, fish, steak, or pork, broiled with no sauce. Ask for a plain baked potato or rice. Avoid mashed potatoes. Ask for grilled or steamed vegetables. Always ask them to leave the croutons off the salad and put the dressing on the side.

Ranch, bleu cheese, or oil and vinegar are okay on my salad. I have even carried salad dressing from home in a small container (I put the container inside a baggie so if it leaks it doesn't cause a mess in my purse.)

But I definitely use a spoon and measure out the dressing onto the salad. Hidden fats in dressing are an easy way to grab some extra calories and disrupt your plan to lose or maintain weight.

Restaurants often post the pre-cooked weight of meats on the menu. They lose a little in cooking. That can be a good guide to ordering. If it is a very large portion, ask for a container as soon as the food arrives. Cut off what you are not going to eat and put it into the container before you start to eat your meal. If doggie bags are not appealing to you, cut away what you are not going to eat and push it to one side of your plate or put it on the bread plate. It is much easier to be mindful of your eating when you do that.

You can stick to a food plan no matter where you go. I have been to Jamaica, Paris, and Las Vegas as well as on ocean cruises and toured the eastern coast of this beautiful country in our motor home. You can eat mindfully anywhere if you set your mind to it.

Chapter Twelve
How Do I Do This At Work

Work presents it's own set of challenges. How can it be possible to eat mindfully in your average office? Well, fail to plan and plan to fail. I am living proof that you can stick to your plan at work. It's the same as sticking to your plan anywhere else, you have to want to do it.

So, what are your problems on the job? First, do you need to clean out all the goodies from those desk drawers? I support you in that. And if you have a candy jar on your desk for others, while you are getting used to the new way of eating, it might be a good idea to get rid of that too. It may not need to be forever, but just until you know that your little fingers aren't going to be dipping into it.

"It's not my food," was a great new motto for me when it came to candy on other's desks. In the beginning of following a new plan like this, it may seem like somebody turned up the volume on all food, but especially what's in the office. Look at all the emotional eating triggers that can occur there because stress is a huge factor in impulse eating for so many of us. But you don't have to eat over stress; it is not a solution. It adds to your problem

What I've discovered about candy is that it gives me an immediate momentary rush of energy, followed by a quick drop in energy. Ever feel like by midday that you need a nap? Could it be that chocolate you've been munching down on?

Giving up the sweets at work is an obvious. If you work with supportive people, you may want to share what you are doing with them. There can be well-intentioned sabotagers who may frequently tempt you. Just remember, "No," is a complete sentence. You do not have to eat for anybody but yourself.

If your office does those covered dish get togethers, in the beginning it might be a good idea to bring your complete lunch with you. Participating is still a nice idea, after all it's good to be social. Just bring something along for the group that you can eat too, like cut up veggies with ranch dressing for a dip or a nice salad. As you get more confident with your new way of eating, you can try more creative dishes.

For me, it was helpful to bring my lunch with me in a cooler bag. That way, I had my weighed and measured meals. If you have business luncheons, re-read chapter eleven for ideas about to order in restaurants. Remember, you can follow your meal plan anywhere.

If there is a refrigerator at work, you may keep some staples in there for yourself, such as salad dressing, breakfast dairy products, enough salad for a few days (weigh it before you eat.)

Also, I keep an emergency meal in the trunk of my car. It includes canned chicken or tuna, several small cans of green beans, yellow wax beans, hearts of palm, garbanzo beans. On more than one occasion I've had to resort to that emergency meal. But I planned ahead, so I didn't have to fail.

Holidays at an office can be quite challenging, especially if you are new at this way of eating. A good tip - don't start on the treats.

If you don't start in on Christmas cookies, Easter peeps or Valentine chocolate, you won't have to stop again. A cookie leads to another,

And another

And another.

If you are in a professional environment and have a lot of weight to lose, be prepared to make some investments in your wardrobe. It made me feel terrific to wear smaller clothing. Thrift and resale shops will help you buy new clothes in smaller sizes without a big initial cash outlay.

When something becomes too large to wear you could either have it altered or get rid of it. Keeping larger sizes is a great excuse to return to old eating habits and the larger clothing size. Having one size wardrobe in the closet is great incentive to not start overeating again.

See that? Now work no longer has to be a big deal either. You can ease into a wonderful new way of life and food does not have to be a problem for you any more.

Chapter Thirteen

At Home

If you live alone, this will be a simple. Clean out the cupboards, the refrigerator, and the freezer. Get rid of all the foods that are temptations for you. Throw it away or give it away. If you are worried about the temptation to eat it, have a friend come over to help and support you.

No, you don't have to have a big food orgy before starting on your new plan, to avoid wasting the food. Who's voice is in your head with that wasted food message? Is it your mama?

Whoever, thank it for sharing and get rid of that food. Wasted food is wasted food. It belongs in the trash, not your body.

If you live with someone who does not have a problem with food and pitching their food isn't an option, create a place in the kitchen that is for their special foods that you do not eat. At our house it's the top shelf of the pantry. There you'll find the microwave popcorn, peanuts, cookies, chips, candy — whatever David wants that I don't eat.

We have a second fridge in the sun room and Dave's stuff is it there too. I have some foods out there, but it is used less frequently and I don't have to look at his food or spend too much time thinking about it. If you don't have the luxury of two refrigerators, make a special place in the refrigerator too.

If you are the grocery shopper, in the beginning you may ask your house mate to buy their own snacks for a while. Today I can buy whatever we need for our family. When the grandkids were here for the Easter, I was able to get candy for their baskets. You see, it isn't my candy any more. It's theirs.

If it seems like you are having to change every thing and that you are putting more focus on food, don't worry. It gets easier. It gets better. Today I hardly think about eating in between meals. I plan what I'll be eating ahead of time and when meal time rolls around, I eat and am done with it again until the next meal. But in the beginning you will have to put more focus on what you are doing. You are changing lifestyles. You're getting rid of the old reflexes.

Like I mentioned earlier, I stopped eating in front of the television for a while. Well, it was more like five years. But that is what it took for me. If you have a history of snacking in front of the boob tube, it might take a while to break that association.

It is good to sit at a nicely set table for your meals. Pamper yourself. Serve beautifully and deliciously prepared meals on nice china. Use cloth napkins. No paper or plastic anything. Play some soft background music. Light some candles. Spoil yourself.

When I became mindful of eating, I learned I practically inhaled food, so slowing down was a huge awareness for me. Try placing your fork down in between bites. Chew. Swallow. Then pick up the fork again. Try to make a meal last at least twenty minutes. Your body needs that long to get the signal to your brain that it has enough to eat. Eating fast does not give you that sated sensation. For me, eating quickly contributed to overeating.

Popcorn was a really big binge food of mine. I had a hard time when David ate microwave popcorn because the aroma filled the house, and I really, really wanted some. So I asked him if he could please not eat that while I was home. Thankfully he honored my request. I think that maybe now I'd be okay if he wanted to pop some popcorn, but if it is too tempting, I can always take the dog out for a walk, right?

When preparing your meal, no BLTs. That isn't the sandwich, it's bites, licks, and tastes. Amazing how much tasting I used to do, and that can add up to a lot of extra food. When it goes into your mouth, it counts. Period. And you are reading the words of a woman who used to eat raw cookie dough. Sometimes there would be no cookies. So watch out for the BLTs, okay?

This is all going to seem hard and time consuming in the beginning but once again, hang in there, it gets easier.

Chapter Fourteen
The Grocery Store

In the beginning shopping can be a harrowing experience. You may think, "How do I shop to stay on a food plan?"

Well, first of all, I stay out of the aisles where I have no business. I don't window shop in the bakery or the aisles where candy, cereals, crackers, rattly bags, and alcoholic beverages are sold. That still leaves plenty of selections for me.

Before going to the store, I think about what is coming up that week. Will I be carrying my lunch to work? Will we be eating most meals at home? Variety has always been a big key to unlock the door to permanent weight loss for me. Generally pre-planning the week's meals will help me have a better idea of what is needed from the store. You may even want to write out your whole week of meal plans before shopping. Whatever is easier for you.

I like doing most of my cooking for the week on one or two days. So I buy large packages of chicken breasts, chopped meat, or beef. Or I might get a large pork, lamb or beef roast.

In the produce section, select beautiful, colorful vegetables for your salads and lunches. I eat raw veggies for lunch in a finger salad by cutting up vegetables so I can just eat with my fingers. I buy for color, texture and flavor. Cherry or grape tomatoes, celery, baby carrots, snow peas, cucumbers, radishes, sugar snap peas, sun-dried tomatoes, bok choy (delicious raw), and snow peas, as well as red, yellow, orange, and green peppers. All are wonderful to eat on the run.

I also like to get some canned veggies too, like hearts of palm, artichoke hearts, and water chestnuts. They really add some zip to that lunch bowl.

For salads, I like romaine lettuce because it keeps much longer than iceberg. Tastes better and has more nutrients. I love to buy spring onions, radicchio, sprouts, and fresh herbs such as arugula, basil, and cilantro to add to salads. The spring mix is nice, but that lettuce doesn't keep like the romaine. Iceberg can be handy to make lettuce wraps for lunch.

When it came to buying prepared foods, I had to learn to read labels. No sugar, flour, or wheat for me. Did you know that soy sauce has wheat in it? I do have that occasionally, but I have to accept that it will make my ears ring more than normal.

Sugar has a multitude of names. Stevia is a safe bet for sweetener, as is saccharin. Many of the others have maltodextrin in them ... that's another one of sugar's nick names. Aspartame has become a popular sugar substitute, but a friend told me that it might be an irritant to my bladder. I had been getting up every two hours to use the bathroom during the night. Since I stopped using aspartame, I no longer have that problem.

I only buy salad dressings when sugar is the fifth or lower ingredient. Watch the low fat dressings as the sugar is higher. You can select a nice olive oil and vinegar too.

Ricotta and cottage cheese, I select low fat. I purchase large eggs and skim milk. The only cereals I buy are oat bran, grits, and oatmeal so I don't have to worry about sugar there.

Most important, read labels. If you see new, improved flavor on the box, it usually means more added sugar, flour, or grease to improve the flavor. So even if it is a product you buy often, read the label.

And don't go to the store if you are hungry. That is the easiest way to impulse buy that I can think of. Have a list. If there is a sale on something that is not on your list, that's okay if it is something you can freeze or has a good shelf life. Avoid over-buying on perishables. Our mothers did a great job warning us about wasting food. If you want to eat it so it doesn't get wasted, forget about losing weight. Just doesn't work that way.

Oh, most frozen vegetables and fruits are okay too, but again, read the labels to check for ingredients you do not eat.

If any food I have suggested here is a binge food for you, don't buy it. Your honesty in this area will be a large determining factor on whether or not this way of eating will work for you.

Chapter Fifteen

Abundance -
Where Do You Want It?

Abundance. I truly believe it is available for every one of us, all of the time. Depends on where I want it.

Prior to 1993, my life was centered around food. I was out of control with food. It controlled me. This was hard to admit to myself. Really, food was deeply intertwined in my daily life. Here's an example of a typical start to my day:

- Get up
- Slowly put my feet on the floor and try to rise gradually until the stinging in my feet from bone spurs subsided
- Enter the bathroom – weigh myself
- Use the toilet
- Weigh myself

- Take off my robe
- Weigh myself
- Maybe take a shower, maybe not
- Check my teeth, if they look dirty, brush them.
- Go out to the kitchen and fix breakfast. *Note*: Breakfast was often affected by what the scale said. If I had lost weight that gave me permission to chow down. If I had gained weight, I may be more determined than ever to stay on my diet, or think, "What's the use? I'm never going to lose weight anyway."
- Eat
- Go back to the bathroom and weigh myself again

Is this any way to start a day? That was my morning routine. The scale was all powerful back then. There wasn't any rhyme or reason to my thinking or the actions I took as a result of weighing myself.

Throughout the day, food or dieting was the main focus. There was a period where I exercised every morning with a trainer, using a stationary bike for an hour at a very high level. My knees hurt so badly that I feared they'd give out on the way to the locker room.

Then I'd stop on the way to work and buy a dozen fat-free muffins at this restaurant called the Old Mill. It's closed since, probably went out of business when I stopped eating there. I was barely out of the door when that box was opened, and I was in it. It was about a three-mile drive from there to the office. I could often eat half the muffins before reaching the office parking lot. Only six could go in with me. If I didn't eat six, they'd wait on the car seat for me after work.

"Here, I brought us each a muffin," I said as I came through the door. My co-workers were beautiful, trim women and one normie man. They'd sometimes eat half a muffin and often none at all. Good. More for me. And then I'd have to sneak them when I thought no one was looking. Any cream cheese or butter didn't count if it went onto a fat-free muffin.

There was also lunch with clients on my expense account. Any way to get more food. And free food was even better. When making sales calls, after visiting a client, there would be a stop at a McDonald's for a Big Mac, large fries, and a milkshake. Then another client and Burger King. I sometimes went to three fast food places in one day. I jammed all the bags and wrappers underneath the front seat of my car.

There were extra trips to grocery stores for my night-time binge stash. Money was no object. I'd stumble into bed many nights in terrible physical pain. Sometimes I'd have a couple of drinks so I could get sick and vomit. Then I could keep eating.

Abundance? I had it all right. Abundance in my mouth and on my body.

I've traded that abundance in my mouth for abundance in my life. There is so much more time for living today, now that food doesn't dominate a large portion of my day.

Now my day starts like this:

- Alarm goes off and I roll over and kiss my sweet husband.
- Get down on my knees and pray. I ask God to be of service to Him that day, for help to remember that food is not a solution to my problems.
- Get dressed and take the dog out.
- Shower and brush my teeth.
- Make coffee and bring a cup and the paper in for my husband (if he's still in bed).
- The night before, I had written the menu for that day, so I prepare the breakfast that is in the plan.
- I read a meditation book and spend some quiet time meditating on what I read.

Then I get into my day, full of life and living. I was able to retire from a twenty-five year management career. My days now are spent coaching, writing, and living a fantastic life.

Abundance in my life. What a trade off. And what a life it is. My husband and I bought a beautiful motor home, and we try to get away for weekends as often as possible. That is a great way for me to travel, bringing along my own kitchen and food.

We went to Paris a few years ago. I stayed on my plan of eating. It was easy. I learned how to say, "no sugar" in French. Most of the menus were in English and French, so I knew what I was getting.

David enjoyed all the wonderful French pastries. I learned that aroma and taste are two separate senses, and that I could enjoy the fragrance of croissants, crepes, and rich sauces without putting them in my mouth. That was so freeing for me. I am not one of Pavlov's dogs. I can separate smell from taste and appreciate both.

Dave proposed to me on a Disney cruise. As we watched the sun set over the Atlantic Ocean, he popped the question. I was stupid in love with that handsome man; I was not focused on the midnight buffets. In fact, when I explained my diet restrictions to the wait staff, the food was prepared exactly to my needs with nothing that was off-limits.

We honeymooned in Jamaica. Was that ever fun. Once again, food was not a problem because it is not the main focus of my life any more. We danced in the moon light, scuba dived off colorful reefs, and climbed a waterfall on the side of a mountain in Ocho Rios. We took naps in hammocks, went horse back riding, and simply enjoyed each other's company. Food was not the focus of our honeymoon.

Remember that 1987 Pontiac Fiero I had to trade in because my fat tummy no longer fit comfortably under the steering wheel? Today I drive a sporty little two-seater Honda S2000. And a motorcycle. When I turned fifty, a bunch of girlfriends got together and purchased the Richard Petty Driving Experience for me, and I drove a real NASCAR race car at 118.1 mph. Thanks to my plan of eating, I was small enough to get in and out through the window of that car. Wowie, wow, wow. I cannot find the words to properly explain how that felt.

111

I can comfortably scuba dive today. The feeling of weightlessness and neutral bouyancy is amazing. I did dive while morbidly obese, but it was a painful experience to get into the water. I needed nearly 40 pounds on my weight belt to get below the surface. Add that to my large body and the fifty pounds or so of other equipment, and there I was attempting to get off the boat at well over three hundred and fifty pounds. I could hardly stand up.

Getting back on the boat was feat in itself, adding the weight of my wet gear to the mix. As you can imagine, I did not dive that much. The weightbelt today is around twelve pounds. Big difference. There is no pain associated with diving. Now I don't even think about the pain. Instead, I can enjoy the wonder of coral reefs and colorful marine life.

Want to trade the abundance in your mouth for abundance in your life? Start today. I don't think I could have it both ways. I had to get away from the excess food in order to find a full life for myself.

Chapter Sixteen
99 Alternatives To Eating

If it is not mealtime and you are wanting to eat, remember that excess food is a one-way ticket to becoming overweight, risking the possibility of morbid obesity. Here are some things you can try instead.

1. Get out of yourself.
2. Have a cup of coffee or tea (no sugar).
3. Drink a bottle of water.
4. Rearrange your bedroom furniture
5. Call your best friend from high school.
6. Clean out a messy desk drawer.
7. Take a yoga class.
8. Make the bed.
9. Dust the furniture.
10. Pay your bills.

11. Read your e-mail.
12. Send a card to an out of town relative.
13. Empty the dishwasher.
14. Call an aunt you haven't talked to in a long time.
15. Clean out your socks drawer, throw away the mateless socks.
16. Start a load of laundry.
17. Take a walk.
18. Ride your bike.
19. Do a crossword puzzle.
20. Read the newspaper from front to back.
21. Take a country western line dance class.
22. Crochet.
23. Watch an old movie.
24. Buy broccoli.
25. Read the manual for your DVD/ VCR.
26. Look up websites for interesting vacations next summer.
27. Learn another language with audio CD's.
28. Pull weeds.

29. Make home-made holiday deco-
    rations.
30. Pray.
31. Meditate.
32. Put on some good music, dance
    by yourself.
33. Flirt with your spouse.
34. Write a letter to your grandkids.
35. Walk the dog.
36. Clean the litter box.
37. Visit a shut-in.
38. Play with your kids on the floor.
39. Write a poem.
40. Play Monopoly.
41. Paint a room.
42. Change the sheets on your bed.
43. Read a good book.
44. Volunteer at the hospital.
45. Dust the blades on the ceiling
    fans.
46. Stretch.
47. Go for a ride in the car.
48. Call an out-of-town family mem-
    ber.
49. Invite a neighbor over for tea.
50. Plan a party.
51. Go to the library.

52. Tell a joke.
53. Get a hobby.
54. Join a committee at church.
55. Offer to baby sit for a neighbor.
56. Plant a garden.
57. Visit a museum.
58. Play solitaire with real cards.
59. Go to a movie.
60. Walk on the beach.
61. Walk in a park.
62. Sew the button that he popped last week back on your husband's shirt.
63. Finish the ironing.
64. Call a friend and tell on yourself.
65. Check the schedule at the local college for that class you've been wanting to take.
66. Hire a coach.
67. Watch *Oprah.*
68. Call in and vote for one of the American Idol contestants.
69. Listen to some classical music.
70. Clean out the vegetable bin in the fridge.
71. Go clothes shopping.
72. Brush the dog.

73. Take up water colors.
74. Visit a nursing home and write letters for the elderly.
75. Scrap booking.
76. Polish your Sunday shoes.
77. Plan a garage sale.
78. Ride a bicycle.
79. Join a local gym.
80. Reconcile your checkbook -- yuck.
81. Write a letter to the editor of your local newspaper.
82. Take a bubble bath.
83. Make a fire in the fireplace.
84. Call your parents and ask how they are doing.
85. Write out your greeting cards for the year.
86. Look at the crazy stuff on You-Tube.com.
87. Take some pictures of sunsets.
88. Go to a local high school sports event.
89. Take all the magnets off the fridge doors.
90. Update your address book.
91. Clean behind the television.

92. Clean the windows, inside and out.
93. Sort through old pictures.
94. Make a God box.
95. Flirt with your spouse ... I know this is on here twice but it's really good.
96. Call your husband/wife at work and tell him/her you love them.
97. Help the kids with their homework.
98. Put new pictures in frames.
99. Read this book ... again.

How many more things can you think of? If you have been using food for a long time to deal with feelings, you may need even more alternatives. Get creative. Have fun. Change your life.

Chapter Seventeen
My Food Plan

Most of us have enjoyed success on one diet or another. But the day comes when we buy into the thought, "one bite won't hurt" and another trip down the over-eating lane commences.

If you have a plan that worked in the past for a while, there's no reason why you couldn't try it again. The key is sticking to it.

But if you want to try what has worked for me, my plan follows:

Breakfast
      1 oz. grain
      6 oz. fruit
      4 oz. protein

Lunch
      4 oz. protein
      12 oz. raw vegetables (finger
            salad)

Dinner
>4 oz. protein
>18 oz. vegetables, cooked
>>and/or raw
>2 Tbsp. fat

This isn't the food plan I've always had. I used to have more carbs -- 4 oz. at dinner or lunch. For a while, I even had a plan with an evening snack. But I've had to change as I got older and need less food. Why is it that we never have to add more food? Heck if I know. But this works for me now.

Let me take that back. I have added food on maintenance. I have another fruit daily, at dinner and I can have rice, potatoes, and other starchy foods now, as part of my vegetable allotment. However, I find I don't eat them very often.

Breakfast Protein
>Bacon, 2 slices (1/2 protein)
>Cottage cheese, 8 oz.
>Eggs, 2
>Ricotta, 4 oz.
>Veggie burger, 2
>Yogurt, 8 oz. (1/2 protein)
>Any item from Protein list

Proteins can be mixed, such as 1 egg and 2 slices bacon or 2 oz. ricotta and one veggie burger.

Breakfast Grains
Ezekiel bread, 1 slice
Oat bran, 1 oz.
Oatmeal, 1 oz.
(Consider adding the following
    on maintenance, but if
    cravings set in, it's best
    to leave them out)
Grits, 1 oz.
Tortillas, 2 soft corn

Proteins
4 oz. of the following(weigh
    after cooking) :

Beef	Liver
Chicken	Pork
Clams	Shrimp
Cold cuts	Sausage
Fish	Sushi
Hot dogs	Turkey
Lamb	Venison

For chicken instead of weighing 4 oz., you can select 2 pieces: breast and wing or thigh and drumstick.

Other Proteins
Beans, 8 oz.
Cheese, 2 oz.
Eggs, 2
Milk, 8 oz. is ½ protein
Tofu, 8 oz.

Vegetables, Raw or Cooked

Alfalfa Sprouts	Greens
Artichokes	Kale
Asparagus	Lettuce
Bean Sprouts	Leeks
Beets	Okra
Beans, green or	Onions
yellow wax	Peppers
Bok Choy	Parsnips
Broccoli	Pickles, dill
Brussel Sprouts	Radishes
Cabbage	Sauerkraut
Carrots	Scallions
Cauliflower	Snow peas
Celery	Spinach
Chard	Tomatoes
Chayote	Turnips
Cucumbers	Water chestnuts
Eggplant	Yellow Squash
Escarole	Zucchini

Starchy Vegetables (limited)

Acorn Squash
Butternut Squash
Corn
Jicima
Peas
Pumpkin
Rutabagas
Spaghetti Squash

Fats

Use two fats daily, a serving is 2 table-spoons:

> Butter
>
> Margarine
>
> Mayonnaise
>
> Oils
>
> Salad dressing
>
> Sour cream

Fruits (6 oz.)

Apples	Orange
Applesauce, no	Peaches
sugar, 1/2 c.	Pears
Apricots	Pineapple
Blackberries	Plums
Blueberries	Raspberries
Cherries	Rhubarb
Grapefruit	Strawberries
Honeydew	Tangerine
Mango	Watermelon

Fresh is best, if canned, packed in it's own juice only.

Bananas and grapes should only be eaten occasionally on maintenance because of their high sugar content.

Condiments

Catsup, sugar free
Herbs, any
Lemon juice
Mustard
Onion soup mix
Salsa
Soy sauce (remember it has
wheat)
Spices, any
Syrup, sugar free
Tabasco
Tomato sauce
Vinegar
Worcestershire sauce

May cook with vegetable, beef, or chicken broth and may consume up to 1 cup a day.

Remember, when in doubt, leave it out. Also, if a food causes a problem for you, don't eat it.

Keeping a Food Journal is essential for me. If I have a day of cravings, I'll make a note on that day's entry in my journal. Then, if I have another day of cravings, I'll go back and look for any common denominators. Look at the sample journal page included at the end of this chapter. It may work for you as is, or you may need to make some modifications. The important thing is to have the journal to help keep you honest.

Some foods may leave you craving something else the next day. I found that when I have caffeinated drinks, I crave volume the next day; I feel insatiably hungry. So it's a no-brainer for me to avoid caffeinated beverages.

Whenever I cook, I'll make enough to freeze some for later. If I am looking for an excuse to overeat, I can usually find one. Part of my new lifestyle is a reversal of that thinking and finding excuses for mindful eating. That is what I do today, eat mindfully.

Daily Journal Sheet Date

BREAKFAST			
	Selection	Weight	Comments
Protein			
Grain			
Fruit			
LUNCH			
Protein			
Raw Vegetables			
Cooked Vegetables			
DINNER			
Protein			
Raw Vegetables			
Cooked Vegetables			
Exercise			
Notes:			

Recipes

The following recipes are flour, sugar and wheat free. Most are pretty quick too, as the majority of us don't have time to spend in the kitchen. I often double recipes and freeze food for another time.

BREAKFAST IDEAS:

OAT BRAN MUFFINS

I love these muffins. They are easy to make and freeze for emergencies.

> 1 c oat bran
> 1 1/2 c powdered dry milk
> 2 tsp. baking powder
> 1 1/2 c egg substitute
> 1 c unsweetened applesauce
> 6 oz.frozen blueberries
> artificial sweetener to taste if
> desired. You can also
> add cinnamon and/or
> vanilla.

Mix dry ingredients, add egg substitute and applesauce. Add blueberries last so the batter doesn't turn blue. Preheat the oven to 360 degrees. Spray muffin tins with non-stick spray and spoon in the mixture evenly to the 12 cups. (don't use cupcake papers, as they stick.). Bake for 20 minutes. Four muffins is one serving. Freeze the other two batches for mornings when you're in a rush.

There's many variations – try adding oatmeal to the oat bran. You can substitute shredded apple and lots of cinnamon for the blueberries.

Please change the measurements for
the muffins to:
1 ½ cup oatbran
1 c powdered milk

PANCAKES

1/2 c oat bran
1/3 c powdered milk
1/2 c egg substitute
1/2 tsp. baking powder
1 or 2 packets sweetener, if
    desired
cinnamon to taste

You can add 6 oz. fruit to the pancakes or serve on the side.

Heat the griddle up and spray with non-stick spray. Spoon the mixture onto the griddle (make 3 or 4). Flip when they are set up, the flip side will be a golden brown. Cook for another minute or so and serve with the fruit and sugar-free syrup.

I LOVE THIS BREAKFAST

1 oz. oatmeal
4 oz. ricotta cheese
6 oz. fresh strawberries

Cook oatmeal with ½ c. water. Add sweetener to taste. Cinnamon also can be used for flavor. Spoon ricotta and fresh fruit on top.

SOMETHING DIFFERENT

1 egg
2 oz. sausage or two slices
   bacon
1 slice Ezekiel Bread
6 oz. sliced orange or
   grapefruit

(when eating out, I've brought the Ezekiel bread into the restaurant with me and asked the wait staff to toast it. I've never been turned down)

APPLE BRAN SOUFFLE

    1 oz.oat bran
    ½ c egg substitute
    2 oz.ricotta
    6 oz.shredded apple
    1 tsp. cinnamon
    sweetener to taste

I leave the skins on but you can take them off if you prefer. Shred apples and place in a microwave safe crock, cover with cinnamon. Bake on high for 4 minutes or until the apple is soft.. Add oat bran, sweetener if you like, and the egg substitute. Cook in microwave for 1 minute. Stir, cook another minute or until center sets. It puffs up like a popover. Add ricotta and some sugar-free syrup if you like.

SWISS CEREAL

> 1/2 c oatmeal
> 1/2 c skim milk (or fat-free,
>   sugar-free soy milk)
> sweetener to taste, if desired
> 6 oz.cut up fruit
> 2 oz.ricotta or 1 c fat-free,
>   sugar-free yogurt

Mix oatmeal with milk and sweetener and refrigerate overnight. Serve the next morning with mixed fruit and the ricotta or yogurt. It's delicious!

BAKED RICE PUDDING

> 1/2 cup cooked brown rice
> 1/2 c egg beater
> 6 oz.grated apple
> 2 packets sweetener or to
>   taste

Mix and bake in microwave four minutes or until apple is cooked through. Center should not be wet. Serve with 1 cup yogurt or 2 oz.ricotta cheese.

PEACH COBBLER

12 oz.sliced peaches
2 oz.dry oatmeal
2 packets sweetener or to
    taste
1 Tbsp. margarine (uses 1 of
    your dinner fats)
1/2 tsp. cinnamon

Preheat oven to 350 degrees. Spray baking pan with non-stick spray. Line with peach slices. In a small bowl, combine margarine, oatmeal, cinnamon and sweetener. Crumble over top of peaches. Bake for 30 minutes. Makes two servings! Top with 2 oz.ricotta or 8 oz.yogurt. Serve warm! Put second serving in fridge for next day.

<u>CROCK POT RECIPES</u>

CROCK POT ROAST BEEF

Line bottom of crock pot with carrots. The baby carrots work well. Place roast on top. You can brown it first on all sides in a skillet on the stove if you like. I've done it either way and it's fine. If you are on maintenance, add some canned potatoes; raw potatoes don't seem to cook through. Add a jar of salsa. Cook on low overnight.

Use the carrots (and potatoes) for your cooked vegetables, weighing out the portion size. Measure the meat.

CROCK POT CHILI

I love chili. There are so many varieties you can make and enjoy. Experiment. Here is one of my favorites:

> 1 lb.ground turkey meat
> 5 cans of beans; mix them up.
> > Black beans, garbanzo, kidney beans, pinto beans ... your choice. 3 Tbsp. chili powder more or less to taste
> 2 Tbsp. cumin more or less to taste
> Sprinkle red pepper flakes, depending on how how spicy you like your chili.
> 1 onion
> 2 Tbsp. minced garlic
> 1 large jar salsa

Brown meat with onions, garlic, chili powder, cumin and pepper flakes. Drain any liquid in canned beans. (I like to use the liquid from the black beans.) Put cooked meat into crock pot with beans and salsa. Cook on low overnight. Great meal to freeze in small quantities for later. One cup is a serving of protein.

CROCK POT CORNED BEEF

Line bottom of crock pot with carrots. Place corn beef on top. Add the little packet of seasoning that comes with the meat if you care to. If you want to add cabbage, you'll need to pre-cook it to el-dente. The cabbage will get that nice corn beef flavor when you add it to the meat. You can also add canned small potatoes. Cook overnight on low.

MEAT, CHICKEN & FISH DISHES

PIZZA CHICKEN

You can use boneless/skinless chicken breasts but I like chicken thighs with skin on. Preheat the oven to 325 degrees.

> Chicken breasts or thighs (or both)
> Low fat turkey pepperoni
> Jar spaghetti or pizza sauce (your choice of flavors, (good rule of thumb, sugar should be 5th or lower ingredient; some brands are sugar-free too)

Place chicken in pan for the oven. Cover pieces with low fat turkey pepperoni. Cover with pizza or spaghetti sauce Sprinkle with some grated cheese. Bake for about 30 to 40 minutes or until cooked all the way through. Don't forget, make enough to freeze some.

MEXICAN CHICKEN

You can use boneless/skinless chicken breasts but I prefer chicken thighs with skin on. Preheat the oven to 325 degrees.

> Chicken breasts or thighs (or both)
> 2 cans black beans
> (when on maintenance, also add 1 cup cooked brown rice.
> 1 jar salsa (use mild if you're not a spice lover, medium or hot if you are)
> fat-free or low fat cheddar cheese

Place chicken in the pan, cover with black beans and salsa. Bake about 30 to 40 minutes or until chicken is cooked all the way through. Turn off oven and sprinkle with shredded low fat or fat-free cheese. Wait about 10 minutes for it to melt. Make plenty for the week and some to freeze. You can use a cup of the beans for a protein too; it's delicious.

CHICKEN WITH SPAGHETTI SQUASH

4 strips bacon
1/2 onion, chopped in large
    pieces
1/2 pepper, chopped
1 stalk celery, chopped
1 c fat-free sour cream
1 c chicken broth
olive oil flavored cooking spray
8 pieces chicken (I prefer
    thighs but you can
    use breasts or a
    combination)
1 spaghetti squash

Cut Spaghetti squash lengthwise and place face down in a skillet. Add ½ inch of water, bring to boil and then reduce heat to medium/low. Cook until the squash is soft and pulls away from the shell. (about half an hour)

Next, in a large skillet, cook the bacon until it is crispy. Remove from pan and add onion, celery and pepper. Cook until veggies are tender. In a blender or food processor, blend mixture with the sour cream and chicken broth. Set aside.

Spray a skillet with cooking spray and add chicken pieces. Cook on medium heat until meat is done. Reduce heat, add blended mixture. Simmer on low heat for 30 minutes.

Measure squash and serve with two pieces (or 4 oz.) chicken and the sauce.

TARRAGON CHICKEN WITH VEGETABLES

> 1/2 c white vinegar
> 2 tsp. soy sauce
> 1/4 c vegetable oil
> 1 tsp. minced garlic
> 1 1/2 tsp. chopped fresh
>   tarragon
> 4 to 6 pieces chicken
> 6 carrots, cut into chunks
> 2 yellow squash, cut into
>   chunks
> 2 zucchini, cut into chunks
> 1 large onion, cut into chunks

Combine vinegar, oil, soy sauce, garlic and tarragon. Reserve ¼ cup. Place chicken and marinade into a large baggie, seal and refrigerate for 1 to 3 hours, turning bag several times.

Drain chicken and place in a baking dish. Preheat oven to 375 degrees. Toss vegetables in reserve marinade and place around the chicken. Bake for 30 minutes or until chicken is tender and no longer pink when tested with a fork. Vegetables should also be tender.

SPICY MUSTARD GRILLED CHICKEN

8 pieces chicken
1/2 c spicy brown mustard
3 Tbsp. . vinegar
1 tsp. olive oil
1 tsp. minced garlic
1/4 tsp. crushed pepper
flakes
1/2 tsp. thyme
3 stalks green onion, sliced

Mix mustard, vinegar, oil and spices together. Pour into a large baggie with the chicken pieces and refrigerate for 4 to 6 hours. Turn the bag several times to marinate evenly.

Preheat grill. Place chicken on grill, skin side down. Use medium heat and cook 25 to 30 minutes until cooked through. Sprinkle with the onion before serving.

LIME AND GINGER CHICKEN

1/2 c lime juice
2 tsp. grated fresh ginger
3 tsp. minced garlic
1/4 tsp. dried red pepper
    flakes
4 to 6 chicken pieces
olive oil flavored spray
1/2 c salsa

Combine lime juice, ginger, garlic and pepper flakes in a large baggie. Add chicken and marinate 2 to 4 hours, turning bag several times.

Heat a non-stick skillet and spray with cooking spray. Place chicken in skillet and cook 15 to 20 minutes or until cooked through. Serve with salsa and lime wedges, if desired. This can also be grilled instead of cooked in a skillet.

CHICKEN AND VEGETABLES

> 6 or 8 pieces chicken
> 2 green, yellow or
>   orange peppers (or
>   combination)
> 3 onions
> 6 to 8 large carrots, peeled
> 10 oz.package mushrooms
> 4 large celery stalks
> 1/2 tsp. each of sage and
>   thyme
> 1/4 tsp. basil
> salt and pepper to taste

Chop vegetables in large pieces. Spray roasting pan with no-stick spray, Place chicken in pan and brown on both sides. Add vegetables. Sprinkle with seasonings. Cover and cook for 45 minutes on low heat. If it starts to stick, add ½ cup water. An an 8 ounce salad makes this a complete meal.

CHICKEN STIR FRY

2 to 3 chicken breasts
1 onion
8 oz.mushrooms
2 stalks celery
1 c bean sprouts
1/2 c pea pods
1/2 c water chestnuts
1/2 green pepper
1 c thinly sliced carrots
1 medium zucchini and
whatever other veggies
you like in a stir fry
1 tsp. soy sauce
1 Tbsp. minced garlic

Cut chicken in thin strips. Spray skillet with canola oil flavored cooking spray. Add garlic and chicken. Stir frequently and remove meat when cooked. Add chopped vegetables and soy sauce and cook on medium heat until veggies are desired tenderness. Measure your vegetables and chicken. If you are on maintenance, you can add 1/2 cup rice in place of 4 oz.vegetables.

CHICKEN PAPRIKASH

4 chicken breasts or 8 thighs
1 tsp. minced garlic
1 paprika
1 c chicken broth
1 c fat-free sour cream
salt and pepper
1 large onion
2 c broccoli (fresh is better. If
        you use the stems, peel
        and cut into chunks
        with the florets)

Season chicken with salt and pepper. Heat skillet on medium and coat with non-fat cooking spray. Add vegetables. Mix chicken broth and sour cream. Pour over top of meat and vegetables. Turn heat to low and simmer for 30 minutes or until chicken cooked thoroughly and broccoli is soft.

ROAST LEG OF LAMB

1 leg of lamb or lamb roast
fresh rosemary sprigs
1 Tbsp. minced garlic
salt and pepper

Score lamb & insert minced garlic and sprigs of rosemary. Salt and pepper. Bake in oven at 350 for about 20 minutes per pound. Check for desired doneness and serve 4 ounces. Good idea to freeze some in 4 oz.packets for a day when you're in a rush.

LETTUCE WRAPS

> 4 oz.tuna
> 2 Tbsp. fat-free sour cream
> Weigh vegetables to equal 12 oz
> Include:
>> 4 lettuce leaves
>> shredded carrots
>> diced water chestnuts
>> sliced tomatoes
>> slivered onions
>> and any other veggie that you
>> enjoy raw

Mix tuna and sour cream. Add seasonings that you enjoy, such as parsley flakes, garlic powder, paprika, dried mustard, or curry. Place tuna mixture and other vegetables in the lettuce leaves equally. Roll up and enjoy your sandwiches! You can substitute tuna with shrimp, crab or other favorite fish.

SKEWERED TUNA AND VEGETABLES

1 lb.tuna steak
green pepper, cut in large
        pieces
cherry tomatoes
zucchini and yellow squash,
        cut in large chunks
onion cut into chunks or little
        cocktail onions
1 bottle salad dressing;
        Italian, Caesar, low
        fat is the best. I like
        the sun-dried tomato
        dressing by Kraft

Skewer fish and vegetables, alternating for color. Place skewers into a freezer storage bag. Add 1 bottle of dressing. Marinate for 3 or 4 hours. Remove and place on a hot grill. Cook until vegetables are tender. Remove from skewers to serve. Weigh out 4 oz.fish. Serve over top of weighed vegetables and compliment with a nice salad.

Also good with scallops, chicken and/or shrimp.

GRILLED MAHI-MAHI

Spray mahi-mahi with olive oil non-fat spray. Season with salt, pepper and paprika. Heat skillet to medium high, spray with non-fat olive oil spray. Place fish on hot skillet. Grill for 2 to 3 minutes, flip and grill on other side for 1 to 2 minutes.

Try not to overcook the fish, as it gets dry. Serve over a really great salad.

SALMON WITH CAPERS

2 lb.salmon fillet
olive oil flavored non-fat spray
3 Tbsp. capers
1 tsp. garlic
lemon pepper seasoning
1/2 c sour cream
1/8 c lemon juice

Spray skillet with olive oil non-fat spray. Add garlic and cook for 1 minute. Lemon juice and capers and cook for another minute. Turn heat to low and add sour cream. Cook for about 5 minutes on low. Coat another pan, coat with non-fat spray and heat to medium high. Place salmon on hot griddle for 4 or 5 minutes, turn and cook on the other side to your desired done-ness. Rare for sushi grade is my preference but if you like it more done, cook until desired doneness. Serve 4 ounces with a little of the sauce drizzled on top. Nice entree for guests or meals throughout the week. Salmon is good cold on a salad.

WASABE SALMON

    4 salmon sashimi grade fillets
olive oil flavored non-fat spray
Cajun spice
1 Tbsp. wasabe powder
1/2 cup cream sauce (see
      recipe in vegetable
      section)

Heat skillet to medium high and coat with olive oil. Sear salmon on both sides. In a saucepan, heat cream sauce and add powdered wasabe. Mix thoroughly and serve on the side of the salmon. Great with Grilled Chinese Cabbage and Mushrooms.

COFFEE-BRAISED ROAST

4 to 5 lb. beef roast
3 cloves garlic (or 3 Tbsp.
    minced garlic)
1 c vinegar
2 Tbsp. olive oil
2 c strong decaf coffee

Put slits in the roast and insert garlic. Place the roast in a bowl and cover with vinegar, refrigerate for a day, turning meat several times. Remove and dry.

In a large skillet or soup pot, heat oil and brown the meat. Pour coffee over top, cover, bring to boil and simmer for two hours or until meat is well cooked. This can also be cooked on low overnight in the crock pot.

STUFFED PEPPERS

> 5 oz.raw ground beef or turkey
> (cooks down to 4 oz)
> 1 large or two medium green
> peppers
> 1/4 c tomato sauce
> 1/2 c mushrooms, sliced thin
> 1/4 c slivered onions
> 1/4 tsp. garlic

Mix ground meat with other ingredients. Cut the top off the pepper and core it. Add mixture. Place in baking pan with a little water on the bottom and bake at 350 for 30 minutes or until pepper is soft. Hint, make four at once and freeze a few. Serve with a 12 oz.salad for a complete meal.

ITALIAN SAUSAGE

> Large package Italian sausage
>   (sugar-free)
> 2 small or 1 large eggplant,
>   cut into chunks
> 2 green peppers, cut into
>   chunks
> 12 oz.package mushrooms,
>   sliced thick
> 2 large onions in chunks
> olive oil flavored spray
> 1 jar sugar-free spaghetti
>   sauce

Spray large skillet with olive oil spray. Cook sausage on medium heat until brown on all sides. Add vegetables and cook until tender, about 20 minutes. Add spaghetti sauce and simmer on low heat for an hour. Serve over cooked spaghetti squash. Delicious!

PORK AND SAUERKRAUT

> 4 to 5 lb.pork roast
> large can sauerkraut
> 1 apple

In a large pot, spray with no fat cooking spray. Brown pork roast on all sides, Add sauerkraut and chopped apple. Bring back to a boil. Simmer for 2 or 3 hours until pork falls apart with a fork.

LUNCH SPANISH OMELETTE

> 1/2 c egg substitute
> 1 oz.ham, chopped fine
> 1/2 oz.cheddar cheese
> 12 oz.raw vegetables,
>   including onion,
>   mushroom, tomato,
>   peppers, chili's
> 2 Tbsp. salsa

Spray pan with non-stick cooking spray. Add egg. Season with salt and pepper, garlic salt if you like. Chili powder also tastes good on this Add raw vegetables, ham and cheese. Cook on medium heat until egg sets on edges. Fold over vegetables in center. When done, remove to a plate and pour salsa over the top (you might want to heat it). Complete lunch.

TOFU

TOFU DIP FOR VEGGIES

    8 oz.tofu

    1 Tbsp. ranch dressing

    1/2 packet dry onion soup mix

Blend in a blender and serve with raw vegetables.

TOFU STIR FRY

    8 oz.tofu, cubed

    1/2 tsp. dry ginger

    1 Tbsp. minced garlic

    1/4 c soy sauce

    1 Tbsp. peanut or canola oil

    18 oz.cut up vegetables, including carrots, bok choy, broccoli, water chestnuts, bean sprouts, mushrooms and zucchini. (or use your favorites in addition or instead of those listed.

Heat up a large skillet or wok, add oil, ginger and garlic. Cook until garlic starts to turn brown. Add tofu and cook for five minutes. Add soy sauce and carrots, cook for about 3 or minutes, then add the rest of the vegetables. Cook to desired tenderness.

TOFU AND CABBAGE

1 small head cabbage
2 tsp. sesame seeds
1/2 tsp. dry ginger
8 oz.tofu, cubed
2 Tbsp. soy sauce
1 Tbsp. peanut or canola oil

Chop cabbage into thin strips. Heat skillet, add oil, sesame seeds and ginger. Add cabbage, cover and cook until tender, about 20 minutes on medium heat.

In a separate pan, spray with cooking oil spray and grill tofu with garlic powder until nicely browned. Measure your cooked cabbage and enjoy.

VEGETABLE DISHES

BOB-A-GANOOSH

This is named after my good friend, Bob in Arp, Texas who loves spicy food! This is one of those recipes where you can add all kinds of vegetables that you like. Here's my favorites:

> 1 eggplant
> 1 large package mushrooms
>> (I like baby portabella's
>> the best)
> 2 good sized yellow squash
> 2 or 3 zucchinis
> 1 large onion
> 2 Tbsp. minced garlic
> 1 small jar prepared spaghetti
>> sauce (watch out for
>> sugar!)
> sprinkle red pepper flakes

Dice the eggplant. Slice mushrooms thin. Slice yellow squash and zucchini. Chop the onion. Spray the pan with no-fat spray and cook the eggplant with the garlic first. Add onion, mushroom, zucchini and yellow squash. Add red pepper (more if you like hot food, less if you don't and leave it out if you are a mild veggie eater.) Simmer on low heat until vegetables are soft, stirring occasionally. Add tomato sauce and simmer for about half an hour. Also a good veggie to freeze for later.

CREAM OF MUSHROOM SOUP

2 heads of cauliflower
1 large can broth (vegetable,
    beef or chicken)
12 oz.mushrooms (baby
    portabella's are great in
    this recipe)
1 Tbsp. minced garlic
2 scallions

Cut up cauliflower and cook in the broth until very soft. Experiment with seasonings. A little curry powder will completely change the flavor! Using a food processor or blender, blend the cauliflower with the broth until smooth. If it is too thick, add a little more broth or water.

Mince the mushrooms. In a skillet, saute the mushrooms with garlic until cooked thoroughly. Add finely chopped scallions for about 3 minutes. Add to the cauliflower mixture. And there you have it, soup. Use as part of your dinner vegetables

CREAM SAUCE

I use this to make a nice sauce to compliment vegetables.

> 1 head cauliflower
> 1 small can chicken broth
>> (vegetable or beef may
>> also be used, but it will
>> make the sauce darker
>> in color)

Cook cauliflower in broth until very soft. Blend. You'll want this to be a little thick so gradually add the broth to the blender. Add spices or herbs to make a special sauce for vegetables. Great over broccoli, mixed with a Tbsp. of grated Romano cheese (count toward fat)

NON-PASTA LASAGNA

12 oz.cooked eggplant
8 oz.cottage cheese
6 oz.spaghetti sauce (watch
     for sugar)
oregano, basil and garlic to
     taste

Peel and slice eggplant lengthwise, very thin. Spray griddle with non-fat spray. Spray top of eggplant slices with a little non-fat spray and sprinkle with spices and garlic powder to taste. Cook on both sides until soft. Cool. Weigh out 12 ounces.

Spray a pan with non-fat cooking spray. Layer with eggplant, cottage cheese and 6 oz.spaghetti sauce. Sprinkle top with 1 Tbsp. Romano cheese as your fat. Bake at 325 degrees for about 30 minutes. Makes one serving for dinner. You can double the recipe and freeze half. (Substitute thinly sliced zucchini for the eggplant or use both.)

BROCCOLI WITH ZING!

> 1 large bunch of fresh
>   broccoli, cut into florets
> 2 tsp. minced garlic
> Pinch of crushed red pepper
>   flakes
> 2 Tbsp. of olive or vegetable oil
> 1/4 tsp. salt

In a large skillet, saute the garlic and pepper flakes in oil. Add broccoli and toss to coat, saute for 8 minutes or until crisp tender. Sprinkle with salt.

LEMON ZEST BROCCOLI

2 bunches fresh broccoli
butter-flavored cooking spray
1/2 tsp. fresh grated lemon zest
1/4 tsp. ground black pepper

Steam broccoli about 5 minutes. Drain. Spray skillet with butter flavored spray and add lemon peel and pepper. Add broccoli and toss in medium high heat for 2 minutes Serve hot.

JEAN MARIE'S BROCCOLI
(Recipe by Jean Marie of Guatemala)

1 Tbsp. olive oil
1 large onion
1 head broccoli
1 tsp. garlic
salt and pepper to taste

Coat skillet with olive oil (or use non-stick cooking spray). Cut onion in half and slice thin. Saute onions and garlic on medium until onions are transparent. Add broccoli, salt and pepper. Reduce heat to low and cover. Simmer until broccoli is desired consistency. (Jean Marie likes it a little crunchy. I like it with the broccoli thoroughly cooked)

BUTTERNUT SQUASH PANCAKE
(Recipe by Susan, Melbourne, Florida)

Cook a butternut squash however you cook it, I nuke it until soft.

Cool, Clean out seeds, scoop out squash

Cook sweet potatoes - again, I nuke them (any size portions),

Cool and peel off skin

Mix together. Weigh off your portion of starchy vegetables and set rest aside. Add some cinnamon, sweetener and McCormicks Vanilla Butternut Flavoring. Spray squash/potato mix with butter flavor spray. And finally, add 4 oz.of Ricotta cheese - mix all.

Spray frying pan with non-stick cooking spray, brown on both sides - and then eat and enjoy. This is a dinner meal; serve with salad and/or cooked vegetables to complete your vegetable portion.

PUMPKIN PIE
(Recipe by Rene of Granbury, Texas)

1 15 oz.can pumpkin
1 can fat-free evaporated milk
2 eggs
2 1/2 tsp. pumpkin pie spice
     (use quality spice)
3/4 c Splenda
1 tsp. vanilla
1 dash salt

Stir all together and bake in a pie plate sprayed with non-stick cooking spray at 425 for 15 minuntes and then reduce heat to 350 and bake another 45 minutes

1/6=1 veggie serving. You may want to cut your protein portion down by an ounce to offset the protein in the pie.

TOASTED GARBANZO BEANS

1 can garbanzo beans (chick peas)

Drain garbanzos thoroughly, place on a paper towel to blot up excess moisture.

Spray cookie sheet with non-stick spray. Spray the garbanzos with butter flavor cooking spray, sprinkle lightly with Tony Chachere's Creole seasoning and garlic powder. Bake at 325 degrees for 30 to 40 minutes until crispy. Shake or stir during cooking to brown on all sides. Delicious on a salad or just by themselves. An 8 ounce serving equals one protein.

(Substitute garlic salt and chili powder for spicy seasoning. You can also try curry or any other spice you enjoy)

BRUSSEL SPROUTS WITH PIZZAZZ!

> Large package brussels
>   sprouts, fresh or frozen
> Olive oil non-stick spray
> 1 Tbsp. . caraway seeds
> 1 tsp. garlic

Steam brussel sprouts al dente. Coat skillet with olive oil non-stick spray. Cook garlic over medium-high heat until it is toasted. Add caraway seeds and brussel sprouts and a little water. Cover and simmer for about five minutes, stirring occasionally. Serve with toasted garbanzo beans and a salad for an interesting dinner!

GRILLED CHINESE CABBAGE AND MUSHROOMS

> 1/2 head red cabbage
> 16 oz. baby portabella
>   mushrooms
> 1/2 c balsamic vinegar
> salt and pepper
> olive oil flavored non-fat spray

Remove the core and slice cabbage very thin. Slice mushrooms thin. Heat saute skillet to medium high and coat well with cooking spray. Add cabbage and mushrooms. You want the cabbage a little crispy. Add vinegar, salt and pepper and cook for a few more minutes.

Serve with Wasabe Grilled Salmon.

SALADS

REALLY GREAT SALAD

If you make boring salads, you'll probably get sick of salads pretty quick. You can prepare the main part of your salad to store in the fridge for a few days.

Line container with a paper towel.

Main part of a salad:

> Romaine lettuce, torn in fork
> size pieces (it keeps
> really well)
> Radishes, sliced
> Hearts of palm (canned,
> drained and sliced)
> Carrots, shredded or sliced
> thin
> Red and yellow peppers
> Cherry or grape tomatoes
> Steamed, chilled veggies such
> as asparagus and green
> beans
> Bok choy
> Scallions
> Chinese Pea pods
> Bean sprouts
> red cabbage, finely chopped
> fennel, sliced

Items to add at meal time:

> Spring mix
> Sliced cucumbers
> Radicchio
> Cut tomatoes

Use your imagination, the more flavor and color in your salad, the more apt you are to eat it. Enjoy your foods!

COLE SLAW

> 1 bag chopped slaw cabbage
> 1/2 c white vinegar
> 1 to 2 packets sweetener (to
>   taste)
> ½ c fat-free sour cream

optional additions:

> 1/2 cup finely chopped green
>   and red peppers (makes
>   it colorful too)

In a bowl, mix the vinegar, sour cream and sweetener, Add vegetables and mix thoroughly. Prepare the day before and let sit in fridge overnight. Really tasty.

CUCUMBER SALAD

> 2 cucumbers, peeled and
>   sliced very thin
> 1 small onion, sliced very thin
> 1/2 c vinegar
> 1/2 c fat-free sour cream
> 6 packets sweetener (more or
>   less to taste)
> 1/4 tsp. black pepper

Mix vinegar, sour cream and sweetener in a bowl. Add sliced cukes and onion. Add pepper and mix thoroughly. Allow to sit in fridge overnight for flavors to blend.

FUN WITH FRUIT

FAKE FROZEN YOGURT

    1 c yogurt
    1 c frozen berries

Mix fruit with yogurt, and it freezes up for a cool fruit treat.

SHAKES

    8 oz. frozen fruit of your choice
    8 oz. skim milk
    sweetener if desired

Mix all ingredients in a blender until smooth!

Cranberry Yum

(recipe by Rene of Granbury Texas)

> 1 lb.pkg fresh cranberries
> (grind in food processor)
> 3/4 c Spenda
> 1 three oz.pkg sugar-free
> gelatin dissolved in 1 c
> boiling water
> 1 grated apple
> 1 c drained crushed
> pineapple, in its own
> juice

Chopped pecans, if on your food plan

Grind cranberries and add the sweetener, if desired. Dissolve gelatin in boiling water and allow to cool. Combine cranberries, gelatin, apple, pineapple and pecans. Refrigerate overnight. 1 cup equals 1 fruit

SAUCES

BAR-B-QUE SAUCE

> Sugar-free catsup (sweetened
>   with fruit juice, you can
>   buy it in most health
>   food stores or use
>   tomato paste.
> Vinegar (experiment with
>   different flavors – I like
>   balsamic)
> Worcestershire sauce to taste
> Sweetener to taste

Mix thoroughly.

This is good on chicken or ribs. Coat meat and cook slowly in oven or on the grill.

Chapter Nineteen
So Now What

It's a lot of information, isn't it? Don't panic. You can make these changes and enjoy life in a normal body size without the encumbrance of excess weight. You can live without that constant chatter in your head about the next meal, the next diet, and the next disappointment.

I started out slow. We had to stop the bleeding first, get the eating down to a sane compromise. Three meals a day and no sugar. Can you do that? It will help tremendously.

Keeping a food journal was my next step. This helped me to see, in black and white, what I was doing. If I had a day where the food thoughts were greater, I could look at the day before for a pattern or a specific food that could be giving me trouble. If it happened two or three times, I considered letting that food go for a while.

Then I made the list of trigger foods, the foods where once I started, I could not stop. It doesn't have to be a big list. You can add to it as you go along, discovering new things that may give you a hard time.

Figure out where your help will come from. Declare war on your overeating. Build the army. The choice is yours but keep looking until you find what works for you. Remember the suggestions from the chapter on getting support? Go back and review it. Try one. If it doesn't do the trick for you, try another one. Don't give up. I really think that this may be the biggest key to unlock your door to permanent weight loss. Get help. I asked God for help. If the word God turns you off, that's okay, just find a power bigger than you. Find a power bigger than food to help you. Talk to friends, a counselor, a coach, a minister --someone you are comfortable with.

As the weight starts to come off, try and remember that rule, one bite will hurt. It leads to another and another. It is insidious. "No," is a complete sentence. It may feel awkward at first to turn down some-one's love offering of food. Food isn't love.

Break down those old beliefs that equate diets to deprivation. Your excess weight is depriving you of a full and exciting life. Use the recipes in this book to develop tasty meals for yourself.

Make your life juicy and delicious. What are you waiting for? If food and your weight has blocked you from a wonderful life, time to kick butt and change that forever. Take it slow at first and build momentum. Start with changing your food, adding exercise and changing your attitude along the way.

Thank your head for sharing. Just because you think something doesn't mean you have to act on that thought. You are not Pavlov's dogs. You are not a trash can. Don't put wasted food in yourself. Don't buy into other's well intentioned offers of food you don't need. You can live without Aunt Suzie's special Christmas goodies. Change your thinking.

I want to be here for you. If you email me at lifecoachgerri@aol.com, I will write back just as soon as I can. None of us has to be a victim to food for one more day.

Ask for help in restaurants. Buy a pocket-sized scale if you need to. Read the labels in the grocery store. Make a plan for work, especially if there is junk food there. When I worked away from home, people became aware of how I ate and respected my boundaries. They'll respect yours too.

Remember that we are all entitled to abundance. You get to pick where you want it ... in your mouth or in your life. Believe me, life is much more fun now that I removed the abundance from my mouth and focused on more in my life. This is available for you too. You deserve it.

You can do it. Start today.